The Cancer Prevention Book

"The book is more than instructions or a plan to prevent cancer. It explains not only what to do but also why we should be doing it. By pointing out that many of the causes of cancer can be removed with a little thought, concentration and effort as is shown by the success stories of patients. The clear writing and the simple structure makes this an easily accessible read which educates and enlightens on a subject that, for all its publicity, is still shrouded with mystery."

— Melissa Lee, *South Yorkshire Times*

"If you have ever wondered if it is possible to prevent cancer by changes to your lifestyle—after all, it has been shown that other diseases, such as heart disease can be affected by a change of eating and leisure habits—then this book is fascinating reading. It is positive, upbeat and possible! Yes, you can change the habits of lifetime!"

— Dr. Susan Hotchkies, *My Weekly*

"[*The Cancer Prevention Book*] explains how we can improve our defenses against the disease by cleaning up our act: eating healthily, exercising, dealing with stress and learning to relax."

— Barbara Lantin, *Daily Telegraph*

Dedication

THIS BOOK IS DEDICATED TO ALL THE PEOPLE WITH
CANCER WHOM I HAVE WORKED WITH. THEY HAVE
SHOWN ME THE POWER OF THE HOLISTIC APPROACH
TO HEALTH THROUGH MANY REMARKABLE RECOVERIES
AND HAVE CONVINCED ME OF ITS ESSENTIAL ROLE IN
PREVENTING CANCER FOR ALL OF US.

Ordering

Trade bookstores in the U.S. and Canada please contact:
Publishers Group West
1700 Fourth Street, Berkeley CA 94710
Phone: (800) 788-3123   Fax: (510) 528-3444

Hunter House books are available at bulk discounts for textbook course adoptions; to
qualifying community, health-care, and government organizations; and for special
promotions and fund-raising. For details please contact:
Special Sales Department
Hunter House Inc., PO Box 2914, Alameda CA 94501-0914
Phone: (510) 865-5282   Fax: (510) 865-4295
E-mail: ordering@hunterhouse.com

Individuals can order our books from most bookstores, by calling **(800) 266-5592**, or
from our website at **www.hunterhouse.com**

The Cancer Prevention Book

A COMPLETE MIND/BODY APPROACH TO STOPPING CANCER BEFORE IT STARTS

Rosy Daniel, M.D.,
with Rachel Ellis

With a Foreword by HRH THE PRINCE OF WALES

Hunter House
PUBLISHERS

Library of Congress Cataloging-in-Publication Data

Daniel, Rosy, 1955
The cancer prevention book : a complete mind/body approach to stopping cancer
before it starts / Rosy Daniel, with Rachel Ellis.
p. cm.
Includes bibliographical references and index.
ISBN 0-89793-361-3 (cloth) — ISBN 0-89793-360-5 (paper)
1. Cancer—Prevention. 2. Cancer—Alternative treatment. 3. Cancer—Risk factors.
I. Ellis, Rachel. II. Title.
RC268 .D35 2002
616.99′4052—dc21   2001039723

Project Credits

Cover Design: Jinni Fontana
Book Production: Hunter House and Jinni Fontana
Copy Editor: Kelley Blewster
Proofreader: Lee Rappold
Indexer: Kathy Talley-Jones
Acquisitions Editor: Jeanne Brondino
Associate Editor: Alexandra Mummery
Sales and Marketing Assistant: Earlita K. Chenault
Publicity Manager: Sara Long
Customer Service Manager: Christina Sverdrup
Order Fulfillment: Lakdhon Lama
Administrator: Theresa Nelson
Computer Support: Peter Eichelberger
Publisher: Kiran S. Rana

Printed and Bound by Bang Printing, Brainerd, MN
Manufactured in the United States of America

9 8 7 6 5 4 3 2 1   First Edition   02 03 04 05 06

Contents

Foreword

ST. JAMES'S PALACE

The Cancer Prevention Book is a remarkable testimony to the enlightened vision of Dr. Rosy Daniel. It tells us not only many of the causes and details of how cancer develops, but also describes some of the things we can all do to help prevent cancer in our own lives. The book has been created both because of twenty years of holistic work with cancer patients at the Bristol Cancer Help Centre and the personal pain and distress Dr. Daniel has experienced as an holistic cancer doctor, watching so many lives devastated by the disease which has impelled her to take action.

Dr. Daniel's courageous work with cancer patients has shown us that cancer, one of our most feared diseases, can be turned around or slowed down, even in its advanced stages. She is now taking an even bolder step to try to take on the prevention of cancer in society as a whole. As a longtime Patron of the Bristol Cancer Help Centre, I am so glad that she has taken this initiative to bring the holistic approach to cancer out into the public arena in an attempt to enable us all to experience the health benefits associated with the Centre's approach, without having to become victims of cancer to do so.

Heartened by the results achieved at Bristol and alarmed by the fact that cancer is currently affecting four in ten people in developed countries—and rising—this book represents a really serious attempt by Rosy Daniel to persuade us all to wake up to the gravity of the situation and take personal and collective responsibility for turning the situation around.

Her point is quite simple—if cancer can be stabilized and the prognosis extended by use of the holistic approach to health for cancer patients, why not use this approach to prevent cancer in the first place? She has been so encouraged by the profound transformations in health and happiness she has witnessed over the years at Bristol, that she is now determined to apply this approach "further back down the river" to help many more of us to experience far better physical, emotional and spiritual health while simultaneously reducing our personal cancer risk.

Bristol has based its successful approach on the holistic health principles of working to improve the health of people with cancer at all the levels of mind, body and spirit. Since the Centre's founding in 1980 by the remarkable Penny Brohn and Pat Pilkington, science has begun, step by step, to vindicate their entirely intuitive approach to fighting and healing cancer. The Bristol emphasis on fruit and vegetables is increasingly accepted as part of orthodox cancer prevention, and the importance of the mind–body connection in health is becoming established through the new science of psychoneuroimmunology. Even the art of visualizing positive outcomes during chemotherapy has been shown to extend survival time with breast cancer. But deeper than this, by helping individuals to tackle the question of the underlying state of their spirit, their relationship to themselves and by rekindling their fundamental purpose and joy in living, enormous and often unexpected improvements in health, well-being and quality of life have been achieved.

Recently the science of epidemiologists Sir Richard Doll and Sir Richard Peto has shown us clearly that cancer, in part, is a lifestyle-related disease which is aggravated by environmental pollution. Our Western disregard for Nature, combined with the emotional and spiritual vacuum often caused by twentieth century living has placed us all at very great and increasing risk. It is gradually becoming clear that smoking, poor diet, stress, pollution and sedentary lifestyles are major contributing causes of cancer. Rather like the Sorcerer's Apprentice, we have in some ways been conducting a vast experiment that has begun to go seriously wrong in many aspects of our existence.

Preface

In *The Cancer Prevention Book* Dr. Rosy Daniel has courageously communicated a wonderful body of information for the understanding of cancer and, especially, its treatment and prevention. Dr. Daniel's wisdom, gained from her many years of experience as a physician specializing in holistic medicine, is evident in her balanced focus on the physical, mental, and spiritual aspects of a healthy lifestyle. She makes clear that these are the areas of our lives over which we can have the greatest influence. She integrates this information into a comprehensive discussion of the prevention of cancer, with particular emphasis on diet and nutrition, exercise, stress and stress management, rest, maintaining energy levels, and achieving peace of mind. She addresses both the science and the common wisdom surrounding cancer. She shows us how many of the approaches used to effectively treat cancer actually work.

Dr. Daniel's excellent explanation of the holistic approach to health illuminates how such a lifestyle is helpful in developing an overall sense of wellness. She makes it easy to see how the integration of body, mind, and spirit works to prevent illness. Her discussion of the field of psychoneuroimmunology helps the reader understand the mechanisms whereby issues of the mind and spirit influence the course of cancer and play an important role in its prevention.

She inspires us with her grounded yet optimistic vision of a world relatively free of cancer and her discussion of how that vision can be realized through a shift in consciousness. Part of that shift, as she points out, comes by focusing on a loving, compassionate, and respectful relationship with ourselves first, and then with others.

She shows us how far from our true natures we have roamed with our increased focus on industrialization and technology, compounded by a breakdown of community, family, and relationships in general. She illustrates how the internalization of unhealthy beliefs and attitudes bears undesirable influence on our health. The lack of importance most of us place on achieving true happiness and purpose has contributed to our increase in illness and suffering. However, by illuminating a systematic pathway to building our self-esteem, fulfillment, and peace of mind, Dr. Daniel then shows us how to increase the sense of meaning and passion in our lives, thereby increasing our will—indeed, our desire—to live.

The inclusion in the book of patients' true-life success stories is extremely helpful. These tales give specificity and vitality to many of the book's most important concepts—such as the role of stress, hope, purpose, and meaning in the dynamics of the development of and recovery from disease. We should all be thankful for these patients' generosity and courage in communicating their personal stories to us.

The final chapter gives us important guidelines about how to change at a healthy pace in a manner we can maintain over time. Even when we need to make wholesale life changes for the purpose of restoring our health, Dr. Daniel emphasizes, it is critical that we carefully monitor our state of mind to avoid feeling overwhelmed, so that we can keep joy central in the process of getting well.

The Cancer Prevention Book is a very wise, courageous, and special book for which we can all be grateful.

— DR. O. CARL SIMONTON
Simonton Cancer Center, Pacific Palisades, California

Acknowledgments

I would like to acknowledge with deep gratitude the support of His Royal Highness the Prince of Wales for the work of the Bristol Cancer Help Centre and for his support of this work on the holistic approach to cancer prevention. The example set by the prince in relation to both organic farming and his rejection of genetic modification are a tremendous source of encouragement to all who seek to promote personal responsibility toward the environment and health care.

My most sincere thanks go to Helen Gummer, my editor for the British edition, for originally commissioning this book and for her encouragement throughout the writing process. I would like to acknowledge the vital role played by the *Daily Express* in the UK, and particularly Sue McGeever, in supporting this project and in helping to publicize this important information on cancer prevention. Huge thanks also go to Rachel Ellis, health editor of the *Daily Express* until December 2000, who worked tirelessly with me to improve the original manuscript and make it more accessible to a far wider readership. Special thanks are also due to the Bristol Cancer Help Centre for its support of this project, and particularly to Chris Head, Pat Turton, Helen Cooke, and Caroline Morrison for their invaluable feedback. I would also like to honor the very great contribution made to cancer care by the Centre's founders, Penny Brohn and Pat Pilkington, since the Centre's opening in 1980 and also to honor the role of Jane Sen in revolutionizing the Centre's approach to healthy eating. Her *Healing Foods Cookbook* is a total delight and is just as applicable to the prevention of cancer as to its treatment. My warmest thanks also go to Professor Karol

Sikora and Dr. Victor Barley for supporting and encouraging my role in making the holistic approach to cancer treatment and prevention more widely known and understood within conventional medical circles.

I am greatly indebted to Dr. Stan Venitt, retired emeritus reader in cancer studies at the Institute of Cancer Research, University of London, for his meticulous guidance in the Chapter 1 section titled "What Is Cancer?" and to Sir Richard Doll, professor of medicine at Oxford University, for his expert guidance on the causes of cancer. I was also helped enormously by the work of Professor Gabriel Kune, author of *Reducing the Odds: A Manual for the Prevention of Cancer;* Theo Colburn, Dianne Dumanoski, and John Peterson Myers, authors of *Our Stolen Future;* David Steinman and Sam Epstein, authors of *The Safe Shopper's Bible;* and Suzannah Olivier, author of *The Breast Cancer Prevention and Recovery Book,* all of whom I have quoted extensively.

I would also like to express my deep gratitude to Reg Flower, Angela Burns, Lynda McGilvray, Zoe Lindgren, and Mair Hoskins for sharing in this book their personal cancer stories and their vulnerability. This is not a step to be taken lightly, and their courage is valued immensely because of the extra depth and meaning their examples bring to the work. My most sincere thanks go to the wonderful, generous Sarah Collins and her team of volunteers for the typing of the manuscript, to Katharine Young and the marvelous production team at Simon & Schuster, and to the excellent copy editor Annie Bridges who pulled the work into shape so beautifully.

I am thrilled that the book is now also published in the United States, and would like to thank Jeanne Brondino of Hunter House for her faith in commissioning the American edition; Alexandra Mummery, my American editor, for her kind help and patience; Kelley Blewster for her superb work in converting all the language and references for the American reader; and the production and marketing teams for their superb help in getting this book out to as large an audience as possible.

But most particularly, I would like to acknowledge my heart-felt gratitude for the great patience, constant encouragement, and unfailing support of Danny Kustow throughout the writing of this book—and especially for his help and the help of my wonderful children, Sophie and Elouise, in my retaining my sense of humor!

— ROSY DANIEL

IMPORTANT NOTE

The material in this book is intended to provide a review of resources and information related to cancer prevention techniques. Every effort has been made to provide accurate and dependable information. However, professionals in the field may have differing opinions and change is always taking place. Any of the treatments described herein should be undertaken only under the guidance of a licensed health care practitioner. The author, editors, and publishers cannot be held responsible for any error, omission, professional disagreement, outdated material, or adverse outcomes that derive from use of any of these treatments or information resources in this book, either in a program of self-care or under the care of a licensed practitioner.

Introduction

Today, cancer touches the lives of almost everyone in Western society, and it is a huge, ever-increasing problem worldwide. While the desperate search for a cure and better treatment goes on, it is clear that we simply cannot wait for medical research to provide all the answers. Instead, we must urgently turn our attention to the prevention of cancer through our own active and positive efforts.

Most people are very scared of cancer but seem to think that, apart from quitting smoking, there is very little they can do to reduce their risk of getting the disease. This couldn't be farther from the truth. In the pages that follow, you will learn about many of the causes of cancer and may be surprised to find that, just like heart disease, cancer is primarily a lifestyle-related disease. This means that if we change our lifestyles and habits, we can considerably reduce our risk of getting cancer. Medicine is progressing all the time, and, hopefully, exciting breakthroughs in cancer treatment will occur within our lifetimes. Meanwhile, if we start taking our health and the precious gift of life seriously, there is much we can do to reduce our own risk potential for cancer.

So many of us live our lives in unfulfilled, insecure, stressed states, in a vicious cycle of self-destructive attitudes and behaviors, feeling unsatisfied by the way our lives and relationships are working out. This is often the result of an emotional and spiritual vacuum created through the breakdown of community and family life—or simply by having focused on the wrong priorities long term—while at the same time failing to nourish our personal spirit. Often, loneliness, boredom, fear, and anxiety cause us to find solace in unhealthy food, cigarettes, and alcohol, whose damaging effects are exacerbated by a sedentary lifestyle and extreme stress. Because these self-destructive behaviors are largely to blame for cancer, it is not a huge leap to see cancer indirectly as an emotional or spiritual problem that needs to be addressed at all levels of our being.

Once we find ourselves in low-energy, unmotivated states, we experience a real inertia or sense of "stuckness." We may know what is good or bad for us but feel quite unable to do anything about it. What we need then is a great deal of support and encouragement and, most important of all, to feel good about ourselves and our lives again. Finding a way out of the inertia trap is the essence of the holistic approach to health, which is based on the idea that our health degenerates as a result of spiritual malaise and that the ability to make healthy changes is linked to the state of our body, mind, and spirit. Getting the right levels of emotional support, guidance, encouragement, and uplift to our spirit is really the only way we can make good, sustainable changes in our behavior.

Until now, most health-promotion campaigns have been based on the dissemination of information, but information alone cannot change the state of an individual who feels stuck. By contrast, the holistic approach to health recognizes that it is vital that we work first on our emotional state; to rekindle our energy, enthusiasm, and, most fundamentally, our will to live and sense of purpose. Following closely behind this is the crucial need to develop self-esteem and a protective, nurturing relationship with ourselves. Only then will it be possible to start changing the way we lead our lives.

But first, some understanding is needed of what cancer is, what causes it, and who is at risk. It is also necessary to understand the current situation with regard to conventional cancer medicine and research—and the politics surrounding them—in order to appreciate the urgency of the situation. While this might make for somewhat depressing reading, the aim is to give you the big picture so that you can see how vital it is for you to get involved personally in the prevention of cancer—both for yourself and for society as a whole. The first half of *The Cancer Prevention Book* takes an in-depth look at cancer: how common it is, its causes, its risk factors and how to reduce them, and medicine's relative ineffectiveness at treating the disease. The second half shows the other, more positive side of the story.

Every form of cancer has been shown, on occasion, to regress or even disappear completely from the body, even after medical treatment has been deemed ineffective. This can happen by spontaneous remission (the cancer simply disappears from the body), which can be made more likely by adopting the holistic approach to health in the presence of illness. The process of remission shows that the body itself has a mechanism for dealing with cancer and that cancer need not be the death sentence so many people perceive it to be.

In healthy people, many hundreds of cancer cells are made every day, and they are either repaired or destroyed through the cells' DNA-protective mechanisms or the body's immune surveillance. It is when those built-in mechanisms for recognizing and dealing with cancer cells break down that cancer can develop and grow in the body.

Even in people who have cancer, the body's protective systems work at very different levels of effectiveness. We know this because there are enormous variations in the time it takes for cancer to spread and for a secondary cancer to appear in different people with the same type of cancer. Sometimes, secondary cancers develop within six months or a year of first being diagnosed, while in other cases diagnosis may take as long as twenty years.

While in part this time difference is due to the grade or aggressiveness of the tumor, it is also due to the level of host resistance—the body's ability to fight back. In cases of cancer remission it is clear that the body's defense system has once again become active and effective. Preventing cancer basically involves understanding and building up these defense mechanisms instead of blindly subjecting ourselves to things that destroy the body's ability to cope and stay well.

The Cancer Prevention Book is divided into six chapters. Chapter 1 explains cancer and its causes. If you are less interested in the disease itself but want to find out how to eliminate the main sources of cancer from your life, begin reading the book at Chapter 2. Chapter 3 describes the most common signs of cancer. Treating cancer early is almost another form of prevention, because many cancers, if treated before they spread to other parts of the body, may never cause problems again. It is wise to make yourself aware of cancer's common symptoms so that, without getting overanxious, you can keep an eye on yourself and your family members and know when to insist on a referral for proper tests or when to get a second opinion.

If you want to go straight to the holistic plan for preventing cancer by achieving positive health, start reading at Chapter 4 onward, using the factual material in Chapters 1, 2, and 3 as a reference to dip into as needed.

Overall, the main purpose of *The Cancer Prevention Book* is to put you firmly in control of your life, in a position to achieve excellent health and a greatly enhanced sense of well-being, vitality, and aliveness at all levels of mind, body, and spirit. The key elements of the plan described in this book have been used by thousands of people with cancer who attended the Bristol Cancer Help Centre, many of whom achieved remarkable recoveries. Examples of their stories have been included to illustrate the power of the holistic approach in fighting cancer and the great relevance of this approach to cancer's prevention as well. For this book is not written for people with cancer—it is for those who are cancer free and who want to make sure they stay that way. My book, *Living with Cancer,* which describes the Bristol approach to cancer, is more suitable for anyone who already has the disease (see the Resources section at the back of the book).

Once you have read *The Cancer Prevention Book,* it becomes a question of deciding which are the most important steps to take to make the biggest difference in your own personal cancer risk. As you read through the following pages, try to avoid getting overwhelmed by the sheer number of possible risk factors involved in getting cancer, a few of which you may be able to do nothing about. However, for most of us, there are usually one or two really important things we could change that could dramatically decrease our risk. Keep an eye out for what they might be for you, and then go about setting achievable goals for yourself as described in Chapter 6, "Getting Started."

It is a good idea to see cancer prevention as a long-term project, and to introduce healthy changes bit by bit. Don't try to change everything at once, because you might risk becoming overwhelmed and giving up. Chapters 2, 4, and 5 contain a lot of practical advice about how to make sustainable changes. If you stick to this advice, realizing that nearly all of our "bad habits" represent an emotional need that must be met in another way before we are likely to be able to change, you should be able to succeed without too much difficulty. It is probable that after making these changes you will soon feel far better than you have in a long time. In fact, by taking the necessary steps to prevent cancer you are likely to experience many other health benefits, too.

The advice given in this book is based upon the holistic approach to cancer that pioneered at the Bristol Cancer Help Centre. It is obvious both to the people who have used the Centre's approach to fighting and healing cancer and to the staff who work there that what has been learned about tackling cancer must now be applied to help prevent it.

1

❖

The Big Picture

THE CANCER PROBLEM

The cancer problem has now reached epidemic proportions in developed countries—four people in ten will get cancer in their lifetime, and one in four will die from it. As the Western lifestyle spreads to less-developed areas of the world, overtaking traditional cultures, cancer incidence in those countries is rising to match that of the West. Yet despite fifty years of intensive cancer research and vast sums of money spent, we are achieving a cure in only three of the rarer types of cancer. Only in testicular cancer, some of the leukemias, and some of the lymphomas is cure a realistic possibility. In the four most common cancers—breast, lung, colon, and prostate—conventional medicine can but hope to increase the "disease-free interval" rather than prolong life significantly.

What research does show is how cancer develops in the body, what causes cancer, and how the incidence of cancer varies around the world depending on local cultures and differences in lifestyle. Sir Richard Doll and Sir Richard Peto have done a good job helping people to understand the priorities for cancer prevention. Their research shows that in the West, 81.5 percent of cancer deaths relate to lifestyle factors: 35 percent of cancer is caused by diet, 30 percent by smoking, 10 percent by reproductive hormones, 5 percent by alcohol, and 1.5 percent by physical inactivity. This leaves only 18.5 percent of cancer deaths attributable to external or environmental factors, such as infection, which causes 10 percent; electromagnetic radiation (EMR), 4 percent; pollution (including food additives), 2 percent; occupational exposure to cancer-causing chemicals, such as asbestos, 2 percent; and medicines and medical procedures, 0.5 percent.

This is not the picture most of the public has about cancer. Generally, people are aware of the connection between smoking and cancer, but most would say the second biggest cause of cancer is environmental pollution. A connection between food and cancer is usually linked to food additives, but as the figures show, these are, along with all other forms of pollution, responsible for just 4 percent of cancer deaths.

The commonly held belief that cancer is caused mainly by environmental pollution makes people feel impotent, thinking that there is precious little they can do personally to reduce their risk of cancer. But this belief is wrong. As we can see clearly from the medical evidence, cancer is a lifestyle disease. It is absolutely vital, therefore, that individually, socially, and globally, we tackle this problem head-on and make every effort possible to eradicate it. With a combination of key information about the causes of cancer and, most crucially, the necessary personal support and motivation to change our lifestyles, the cancer picture could be changed dramatically.

For the past fifteen years I have worked as a holistic doctor and, most recently, as medical director of the Bristol Cancer Help Centre. At the Centre, we use the holistic approach to health to help people with cancer fight to regain their health. It has become crystal clear at Bristol that there are many steps that individuals can take to promote their own health, which, even in the presence of illness, can make a crucial difference in their efforts to stabilize the disease. Over the past twenty years many of the people who have undertaken the Centre's holistic approach have undergone a profound revival of their health, happiness, and fulfillment;

frequently they are heard to lament, "Why oh why did I have to wait until I got cancer to come alive and really experience true health in this way?"

Reg Flower was diagnosed with malignant melanoma in 1982 and found his way to the Bristol Cancer Help Centre after stumbling by chance upon an article about the Centre in the paper. He was immensely relieved to be given practical steps to fight his cancer through diet and complementary medicines. But it was not until a year later, when he developed secondary tumors a few months after being abruptly and traumatically laid off from his job, that the deeper value of the Centre's approach really came home to him. Reg was absolutely devastated by his job loss, as twice he had personally pulled his firm back from the brink of bankruptcy and had been promised a position on the firm's board. He had always been a workaholic, putting everything he had and more into his work, covering up other people's errors or failures. He failed to see how his dedication to the firm could possibly have resulted in termination. He was also very frightened by the recurrence of the disease and realized that something major had to change if he was going to survive.

When he returned to the Centre, the first crucial thing he managed to do was to let go of his characteristic stoicism and express his emotions in counseling sessions. With enough support he overcame a lifetime's inhibition, weeping and raging until his hurt and anger were fully expressed. He then, to his own amazement, having always been a "tough sort of bloke," discovered the profound benefits of spiritual healing, relaxation, and meditation. Within a short while, his perspective on life changed completely. He began to regain his sense of humor, learning to laugh at himself for having gotten things so dreadfully out of proportion for so many years. He just could not believe that he had allowed his work to take him over so completely. He realized what was really important to him and began to put time and energy into being with his wife and children. He started growing organic vegetables in his garden, and spent hours in his garage making rocking horses for the kids, rather than new prototypes for his engineering work as he had before. But even more important, he learned how to take time simply to be with himself or to stop and appreciate the beauty of life around him. He says that after the change in his life, he would stop the car and sit for an hour or two just watching the sun go down—deeply moved by the beauty of nature and his sense of connection to it.

In the years that followed, Reg started his own business and did extremely well, but he was always mindful of the necessity to keep his priorities straight. At this point in 2002, he is still living, nearly twenty years after having had secondary melanoma and being told he had maybe two years more to live, if he was lucky.

Reg is sure that his survival is due to his wholesale adoption of the holistic approach to health and his changed lifestyle. But his great frustration is that people have to get seriously ill to get their lives sorted out in this way. He says, "If only people could do all this before they got ill. All I see around me is miserable-looking people rushing around in ever decreasing circles, stressed out of their minds about some total irrelevancy, making themselves sicker and sicker in the process. Every time I get on the tube in London, I see tense unhappy faces—no one is smiling. If only they could all stop and get back to what really makes them happy and brings them alive. I had to do that, and not only has it saved my life but the pleasure I now get out of the simplest things is mind-blowing. We have to get this message across to people who are still cancer free—for God's sake stop the risky things you are doing and act now to get your priorities right. Learn from those of us who have trodden this path before you. We've been through it and learned the hard way—you don't have to do that if you follow the holistic plan now and get your life and health back into shape!"

It has been immensely gratifying to walk this path with many thousands of people with cancer, helping them find their mental, physical, and spiritual healing. But the pain, fear, and anguish caused these individuals by this extremely nasty disease has impelled me to try to help people everywhere to employ the holistic approach to health before cancer develops. I have witnessed so many remarkable recoveries from cancer through the use of the holistic approach that it seems obvious to me that people can also use it to prevent the disease from arising in the first place.

People who come to the Bristol Centre describe cancer as the most shocking wake-up call, compelling them to completely rethink their relationship to themselves, to their health, and to life itself. Surely it is possible for all of us to wake up right now and take stock of the state of our lives, health, and well-being—*before* we are terrified into doing so.

The aim of this book is to help those who wish to make radical improvements in their health to identify the factors that are currently compromising them and putting them at risk. The book also provides step-by-step guidance on how to get the right level of support to address and remove these obstacles so that an entirely new state of enhanced physical health and well-being can be reached. Many of us equate getting healthy with assuming a monastic lifestyle in a state of terrible deprivation. This is a great fallacy. In reality, the effects of a heavy Western diet, toxic smoke, alcohol, obesity, inactivity, and boredom cause our minds and energy levels to become extremely sluggish and lead to increasingly deep apathy and unhappiness. On the other hand, the sense of aliveness and exhilaration that we experience as we shed these layers of sedation and toxicity, live out our passion and purpose, and achieve our potential is quite wonderful and could not be more exciting!

In this book you are given the opportunity to:

❖ learn about cancer, its causes, and the current state of cancer medicine and research;

❖ learn about the holistic approach to health and how to clean up your act, eliminating potential sources of cancer from your life;

❖ learn how to maximize your physical health so that you become positively healthy rather than just disease free;

❖ learn to optimize the effect that your mind, spirit, and lifestyle have on your physical health.

Throughout the book, emphasis is placed on showing how you can get emotional support to make the necessary changes, rather than on merely providing information about the things you need to change. This type of support is crucial to making any sustainable health-promoting change.

Before you embark on this practical step-by-step approach, it is important to first take an in-depth look at what cancer is and what causes it, since this will put all the other recommendations into perspective. However, as said earlier, if you find the technical aspects of cancer too heavy, you can go straight to Chapter 2, which deals with the practicalities of how to reduce the cancer risk in your life.

WHAT IS CANCER?

Cancer is a disease that results from the uncontrollable growth of cells in the body—most commonly due to damage of the cells' genetic material (DNA) or to other abnormalities that stimulate repeated cell division. A cancer arises from a single cell that has become abnormal and that multiplies and multiplies until a solid mass of tissue, or a tumor, is formed. In the case of blood cancers, the blood becomes full of abnormal blood cells. Because there are two hundred different kinds of cells within the body that are the starting point for all our different tissues, there are as many different types of cancer. This makes the study of cancer an enormously complex business. However, the underlying principles of what causes healthy cells to "go wild" and become cancerous are becoming increasingly well understood.

All cells contain a nucleus that contains twenty-three pairs of chromosomes. Each time a new cell is formed, the twenty-three pairs of chromosomes split apart and are copied, or replicated, so that a new pair of each of the twenty-three chromosomes goes off into each daughter cell. All along these chromosomes are genes that are sequences of informational blueprint, or codes, for the manufacture of every sort of tissue and chemical within the body. Cells are dividing and replicating all the time; scientists estimate that in a healthy body, most of the tissues are replaced about every two months. The more dense, bony tissues have a slower turnover rate but are still in a constant state of flux.

DNA Damage

In healthy cells there is an orderly process of replication or copying of the genetic information. In order to do this, the DNA must be replicated exactly, so that the two resulting cells are identical and healthy. The problem comes when errors occur in the replication process. It is estimated that faulty DNA replication occurs in only one in one million million replications, a miraculously low rate! When errors do occur, one of three things can happen. Either the cell corrects the damage, or it becomes so abnormal that it is programmed for cell death, which is called *apoptosis*. The third, much more dangerous thing that can happen is that the changed DNA escapes the cell's repair or suicide mechanisms and is passed to the new daughter cells and to all subsequent generations of cells as division continues. The changes in the DNA that are propagated throughout subsequent cell divisions are called *mutations*.

This very tiny, natural mutation rate of cells within the human body is increased dramatically by exposure of the cells to *mutagens*—substances that induce genetic changes that may lead to cancer. The process is also increased by other tumor-inducing agents or physical mutagens, such as cancer-causing viruses, radioactivity, and ultraviolet radiation from sunlight, as well as by the cells' own toxic waste (the by-products of cellular metabolism). The initial mutation is only the first of five or six mutational steps toward the creation of a malignant cell. We now know that, over time, sequential mutations accumulate in the damaged cell to the point where the cell's growth and repeated division become out of control. At this point, the tumor formed has the potential not only to grow rapidly in the tissue of origin, but also for daughter cells to break off from the main tumor and travel in the bloodstream. These stray cells can then take up residence in other, distant parts of the body, growing there as secondary cancerous tumors, known as *metastases*.

The process by which cancer develops, called *carcinogenesis*, occurs in three stages: initiation, promotion, and progression. *Initiation* is sparked by "initiators" or triggers (usually mutagens), which cause changes in DNA structure. Agents that cause *promo-*

tion are effectively those that pour fuel on the fire, accelerating the growth of cancer cells. *Progression* is the term used for the process by which a benign tumor becomes malignant: Rapid cell growth of fairly normal cells occurs, but over time, the cells begin to turn nasty, eventually becoming a full-blown cancer. Many carcinogens, such as asbestos, are called *complete carcinogens* because they can cause all three processes to occur.

Some carcinogens consistently cause cancer in specific organs. A good example of this is aflatoxin B—produced by certain molds that contaminate staple foods such as grains—which causes liver cancer. Another is asbestos, which causes cancer of the lining of the lung, called *mesothelioma*. Exposure to several carcinogens simultaneously can have a compound effect that is greater than the effect of individual carcinogens. For example, lung cancer is far more likely in a person who smokes and has also been exposed to asbestos.

Mutation

There are three main types of mutation that can either occur spontaneously or can be caused by carcinogens. The first type is a *point mutation,* where one particular bit of the genetic information is changed or deleted. Normally, the genetic code is set in groups of three "letters" or "bases." So if we imagine that the gene information normally reads "Bob got one egg for Jim," the substitution of one letter could leave us with "Bob got one ego for Jim." Clearly, the original sense is lost. This type of *base-pair substitution* accounts for many of the P53 cancer-gene effects that have been well publicized by the media (see the section later in this chapter titled "Tumor Suppressor Genes").

Another kind of point mutation is caused when there is an omission of one letter (or base). By losing the letter *o* in Bob, for example, the other letters move forward and we get "Bbg oto nee ggf orJ im." This is called a *frame shift mutation.* It creates a very distorted genetic message all along the chromosome, just by the loss of one bit of information.

The second type of mutation is called *chromosome mutation*. This happens when chromosomes break and are reassembled in the wrong order. This type of mutation is thought to be of critical significance in cancer. The third type is *genomic mutation*, where there is a change in the actual number of chromosomes in the nucleus. Loss or gain of a single chromosome is known as *aneuploidy*, and this is also regarded as a very important element in the process of carcinogenesis.

DNA has many potentially reactive sites along its structure to which other, harmful chemicals can join. Among these are the dangerous reactive chemicals called *free radicals*, which can be produced within the cell itself as toxic by-products of cellular metabolism. Others include carcinogenic chemicals from the environment (such as polycyclic aromatic hydrocarbons from exhaust fumes and smoke), and many other environmental pollutants that can find their way into the cell nucleus and bind to DNA.

Once bound to DNA, these chemicals are called *adducts*; they play a major role in carcinogenesis. Sometimes the adducts form cross-links between the two strands of DNA, inhibiting proper replication. Adducts can be so bulky that they distort the DNA structure and cause errors during DNA replication. In other cases, due to the presence of adducts (or of different triggers, like X rays), single and double strands of DNA break and in turn can create more free radicals. *Free radicals* are atoms or molecules that contain an unpaired electron that seeks out other electrons from neighboring chemicals to attain a more stable and less reactive state. The free-radical damage caused by this process is involved in several important mechanisms of carcinogenesis, including those caused by chromium, nickel compounds, and asbestos.

We now have a picture of a cell whose DNA has become mutated by an initiator, and that then goes through five or six successive mutations, escaping the normal repair or suicide mechanisms of the cell, producing a new cell line that, paradoxically, has a survival advantage over the cells around it. Very often it is the genes involved in cell repair that mutate, seriously impairing the cell's ability to protect itself. Once this crucial function is lost, the

cell can start to multiply out of control. The most important mutations occur in genes that:

❖ control communication between cells, known as *signal
   transduction;*

❖ control the cell's growth cycles;

❖ maintain gene stability;

❖ mediate cell death, called *apoptosis;*

❖ are normally responsible for controlling the life span of cells.

Normally, the DNA code is checked and corrected by "proof-
reading" systems during and after DNA replication. Once abnormalities are detected, division can be halted and DNA repaired.
This can happen in a series of steps called:

❖ damage targeting

❖ incision

❖ damage removal

❖ resynthesis

It is when these surveillance and repair operations themselves
become faulty that the trouble begins.

Genes that control cell growth cycles and genomic stability
have been identified and found to be mutated in human cancer.
They are often referred to as "cancer genes," a useful shorthand.
However, it must be remembered that a cancer gene is a mutant
version of a normal gene that now creates abnormal proteins itself
or has become lost altogether.

GENETIC PREDISPOSITION TO CANCER

Over the past decade the press has emphasized the new understanding of the inherited risk of cancer and the presence of inherited cancer genes, or oncogenes, as they are known. What must be
stressed straightaway, however, is the current estimate that

between only 1 percent and 5 percent of all cancers come through this hereditary route.

Oncogenes are mutant forms of a large family of genes called *proto-oncogenes*. Proto-oncogenes are genes that normally control cell growth and proliferation, helping to see cells safely through their normal growth cycle. When they become mutated, they become dangerous because they fail to work effectively at monitoring cell growth.

Tumor Suppressor Genes

The other side of the picture is that healthy cells also contain tumor suppressor genes, which are involved in maintaining the stability of the cells. When these become mutated, cells are able to grow out of control. The best known of these suppressor genes is the P53 gene. It is estimated that probably half of all cancers contain P53 mutations. The P53 gene is easily affected by carcinogens such as aflatoxin B, carcinogenic substances in tobacco smoke, vinyl chloride and chromates (used in industrial processes), and asbestos, as well as by radioactivity and ultraviolet radiation from sunlight.

Germline Mutation

So far, the mutations mentioned have been those that happen within one person from cell to cell as cells in the body divide. This is known as *somatic mutation*. Another possibility, called *germline mutation,* occurs when mutations occur in the reproductive tissues—the eggs in the ovaries or the sperm in the testicles. This makes it possible for mutations, and therefore a risk of cancer, to be passed on to the next generation. The most common inherited defects are abnormalities in the tumor suppressor gene. Such inherited defects are rare, however; the majority of cancers occur as a result of somatic mutations.

Overall, the risk of cancer can be classified by dividing the population into four groups:

❖ a background "spontaneous" group, in which random mutations occur in normal people

❖ an environmental group, in which mutations may be caused by chemicals, radiation, or viruses, or a combination of these factors

❖ an environmental/genetic group, made up of people who are at greater risk from exposure to carcinogens owing to what are called *pharmacogenetic polymorphisms*, which means they break down certain chemicals in a more dangerous way, creating by-products that are toxic to the body

❖ a purely genetic group, in which genetic susceptibility is more important than either spontaneous or environmentally induced events

Screening for DNA Damage

Genetic science has moved so fast that the entire human genome, which determines human life, is now completely mapped out. As a result, it is rapidly becoming possible for gene structure to be checked using DNA microchip technology. The whole human genome can be contained on just ten microchips! It will also soon be feasible to assess individuals for mutations in oncogenes and tumor suppressor genes, as well as to check for the presence of pharmacogenetic polymorphisms. Checks like this could alert people to their individual susceptibility to the environmental and occupational toxins that can trigger cancer, thus helping to identify those who are at increased risk. Within our lifetime, this kind of test may become a realistic part of cancer prevention.

In the workplace, it is also becoming possible to monitor body fluids or tissues for genotoxicity and DNA adduct formation (called *biomonitoring*). The aim of biomonitoring is to prevent occupational cancers by giving early warning of exposure. Where occupational exposure does exist, it can be severely compounded by other factors such as smoking, diet, drugs, medical procedures, and other diseases. As with environmental carcinogens, the effect of occupational chemical exposure may be exacerbated if an individual is less able to reduce the carcinogenic threat in the body. Meanwhile, industrial and medicinal chemicals are now routinely tested for their ability to damage DNA, so that dangerous exposure to carcinogenic chemicals is reduced at the source.

It must be stressed that there are also carcinogens that do not damage DNA. These include:

❖ enzyme inducers, which speed up enzyme activity in the cell

❖ hormones (either made by the body, taken as medicines, or from environmental pollution directly or in the form of chemicals known as *endocrine disrupters*)

❖ hormone modifying substances

❖ various chemically inert materials

The common factor in these types of chemicals is their ability to stimulate sustained cell division instead of damaging the DNA itself. The problem is that rapidly dividing cells are more prone to mutation, increasing the risk that cancer may develop.

As people get older, there is also an increase in the frequency of mutation. This may account in part for the greatly increased cancer incidence in older people in comparison with children or young adults. Other important factors in this phenomenon include:

❖ the buildup of free-radical damage in the DNA

❖ progressive failure of DNA repair

❖ the time needed for a particular cell lineage to accumulate the number of different mutations necessary for cancer to develop

THE GROWTH OF A CANCER

Once a cancer cell lineage is established, its cells begin to multiply unchecked. Once the tumor growth passes a volume of 1 cubic millimeter, it requires a blood supply and starts to evolve its own capillary network. Eventually the tumor grows big enough to invade surrounding lymph and blood vessels. And when tumor cells then break off and migrate through the lymph and blood systems, the really serious side of cancer begins.

In the early stages of tumor growth, it is sometimes possible for the immune system to eradicate tumor cells. However, tumor cells can also develop mechanisms to avoid detection by the immune system, allowing the tumor to grow unchecked. When cells reach nearby lymph nodes, the body often attempts to fight back and the lymph nodes swell. Nonetheless, in many cases, the rapidly dividing cancer cells take over the lymph nodes, and the cancer spreads farther.

By this stage, cancer cells will also have entered the bloodstream. These breakaway cells can become lodged in distant capillary beds in key organs such as the liver, lung, or brain, where they can then begin to multiply, forming new tumors. It is at this point that the cancer may become life threatening, because the secondary deposits or metastases can grow large enough to cause failure of the vital organs, severe weight loss, and, in many cases, death.

WHAT CAUSES CANCER?

Based on what we currently know, the main causes of cancer in developed countries, in order of seriousness and with percentage of deaths attributable, are:

- ❖ diet (35 percent)
- ❖ smoking (30 percent)
- ❖ reproductive hormones (10 percent)
- ❖ infection (10 percent)
- ❖ alcohol (5 percent)
- ❖ electromagnetic radiation (4 percent)
- ❖ pollution and food additives (2 percent)

- ❖ occupational hazards (2 percent)

- ❖ physical inactivity (1.5 percent)

- ❖ medical procedures (0.5 percent)

These percentages were calculated by British epidemiologists Sir Richard Peto and Sir Richard Doll of Oxford University in their joint Imperial Cancer Research Fund and Medical Research Council study. The picture created by the findings of these world-renowned scientists shows that cancer is a lifestyle-related disease, with environmental factors contributing only a tiny proportion to overall cancer mortality.

That view is strongly challenged by environmentalists, who believe that the role of intensive agriculture in carcinogenesis, with agriculture's heavy reliance on the use of chemical pesticides and fertilizers, and of traffic and industrial pollution is much higher. Environmentalists also believe that the effects of intensive farming significantly reduce food quality, which in turn influences an individual's susceptibility to cancer because of the lack of key minerals in foods. There is also serious concern about the presence of carcinogens in many common household products we all use daily.

It is vitally important to look not only at what is proven scientifically beyond any shadow of doubt, but also at newer theories that may receive less scientific attention. In some cases, the lack of attention given to a theory may be due to the threat that such research could pose to the livelihood of the farming, manufacturing, petrochemical, drug, and industrial communities.

In describing the process of carcinogenesis, what becomes clear is that it is a complex, multi-step process. We know that there are some agents (such as asbestos) that are so damaging to cell nuclei and genetic material that their influence alone can cause cancer. However, it would appear that in the majority of cancers there is a synergistic effect of several types of factors. It is very likely that the toxic load that accumulates in the body over a lifetime from ingested pollutants, through diet, or by inhalation through the lungs sets the stage for the chemistry of cells to become abnormal. Scientist and professor Sam Epstein, in *The Safe*

Shopper's Bible (see the Resources section), says that over four hundred chemical contaminants have been found in the tissues of humans. Other scientists estimate that "healthy" British women have some two hundred chemical pollutants in their breast milk!

Because of the heavy chemical load on the body, we need to know the status of the body's ability to eliminate toxins, and why this ability seems to have become so compromised. One of the main factors implicated is sedentary lifestyle and obesity. It is interesting to note that physical inactivity is now included among the measurable causes of cancer. The body's cleansing mechanisms rely almost entirely on muscular activity to remove toxic waste from the tissues, and it is entirely understandable that allowing the body to become sluggish and the tissues "stagnant" should result in higher cancer rates. What must also be considered is the fact that many of these chemicals do other damage in addition to their having a carcinogenic effect. They are often directly toxic to the immune cells, breaking down the body's first-line defense mechanism. Many chemicals can dissolve and be stored in our fatty tissues because fat is a universal solvent. Not surprisingly, this problem increases in direct proportion to how overweight we are and how little we exercise.

The Mind/Body Connection

What remains completely unaddressed currently, by both conventional and environmental groups, are the effects our mind and spirit can have on the body's chemistry and immune function and on the development of cancer. Indeed, over the decades much skepticism has been aimed at the notion that the mind has anything whatsoever to do with physical illness. However, in the last twenty years, revolutionary developments in the field of psychoneuroimmunology (PNI)—the study of how the mind and body are linked—have proven categorically that mind and body are inextricably connected.

We are rapidly on the way to understanding how the state of our mind and spirit and the use of mind/body techniques can profoundly affect our body's ability to resist and recover from illness.

When people grow dispirited or crushed, or have lost their way in life, medicine becomes much less effective. Conversely, when they become excited and motivated, living purposeful lives over which they feel they have control, the incidence of serious disease falls and the success of treatment greatly increases. Hard scientific data exist on the role of stress, depression, isolation, and emotional repression in depressing our immune function, and the way these things affect our ability to both resist and ultimately survive serious disease. There is also a wealth of evidence on the role of mind/body techniques and psychological support in improving symptoms, well-being, and survival rates.

A great deal more work needs to be done, however, on the role of stress and distress in decreasing immunocompetence and disease resistance in the West. Such studies will be particularly important in helping to identify those at increased risk of stress-induced illness. Early work shows that some people have a much stronger physical response to stress and unhappiness than others. Just as there are individuals who are more vulnerable to carcinogenic chemicals as a result of pharmacogenetic polymorphisms, it is likely that there are people whose genetic makeup makes them more susceptible to the mind/body effects of stress, distress, and isolation. The jury is still out on this subject. I will begin here with a more detailed look at the proven causes of cancer. Following that discussion, I will present the environmental arguments and then finally will explore the more controversial issue of the role of mind and spirit in cancer causation.

Diet
An unhealthy diet causes 35 percent of cancer deaths.

The Western diet is currently considered the single most significant cause of cancer deaths in developed countries. This may be a great shock to people who believe that smoking and environmental pollution are the biggest causes of cancer. Even those who realize the important connection between diet and cancer seem to think that the cancer-causing elements in our diet are food additives and environmental pollution. The current conventional wisdom, however, is that food additives and pollution cause only a tiny proportion of cancer deaths: It is the ratio of the different elements of fat, sugar, salt, protein, vegetables, fruit, and starch in our diet that is at fault.

Dietary Imbalance

As evidence accumulates, the recurring finding is that it is plant materials known collectively as phytochemicals that protect us from cancer, while excessive protein, fat, and sugar seriously increase our risk. Food processed to its refined state also increases our risk because the processing removes vital minerals, vitamins, and the plant phytochemicals that are so crucial to the body's normal, healthy cellular function. The dangers facing society can be quickly appreciated by considering the fact that children in developed countries are currently estimated to get over 75 percent of their daily calorie requirement from carbonated drinks and sweets. This is a major problem because these foods contain only empty calories with virtually no nutritional value. In the UK, it is estimated that 47 percent of children currently eat no vegetables other than fried potatoes! These statistics indicate that, while children may be getting more than enough energy and calories to function and become obese, the vital nutrients required for healthy growth, immune function, and intracellular protection from cancer are inexorably depleted, and their vulnerability to major degenerative diseases such as cancer is greatly heightened. The resulting vitamin and mineral deficiencies in children can impair their learning ability as well as cause violent and disruptive behavior. Our children are an accident waiting to happen. This nutritional problem in children must be addressed as a matter of great urgency.

Obesity

In addition to the nutritional compromise created by the Western diet, another important factor in the relationship between diet and cancer is obesity. American scientists have shown that when the body mass index rises from twenty-two to thirty-two, there is a 40 percent increase in cancer incidence. Body mass index (BMI) is calculated by dividing your weight in kilograms by the square of your height in meters. (To determine your weight in kilograms, divide your weight in pounds by 2.2. To determine your height in meters, divide your height in inches by 39.4.) For example:

140 pounds ÷ 2.2 = 63.6 kilograms

65 inches ÷ 39.4 = 1.65 meters

$1.65^2 = 2.72$, so BMI = 63.6 ÷ 2.72 = 23.4

It has been noted that in prisoner-of-war camps, women who were more than 10 percent underweight were never seen to have breast cancer. The same finding occurs in animal studies; underweight animals rarely have cancer. This clearly points out that cancer is a disease of affluence.

The cancers most strongly affected by obesity are cancers of the breast, endometrium (uterine lining), colon (large intestine), and gallbladder. The exact reason why obesity is so important is not entirely clear. However, body fat is a major source of estrogen—especially in postmenopausal women—and many cancers are hormone sensitive (i.e., their growth is accelerated in the presence of high hormone levels).

Along with the extra hormonal influence on the body created by obesity, there is another problem connected with fat. Like water, fat is a universal solvent. This means that body fat acts as a storage house for chemical toxins (organic rather than inorganic) that we absorb from our food or through our lungs. Organic chemicals are those that are based on a carbon-ring structure that is found in manmade petrochemicals and plastics as well as in many naturally occurring substances. This fatty storehouse for chemical pollutants maintains high toxin levels in the body, subjecting the cells to long-term unwanted chemical influences. People who eat a diet high in animal and plant fats absorb and store the fats that the animals or plants themselves stored over their lifetime. Humans, because they are at the end of the food chain, therefore get the cumulative effect of this toxic buildup. If we are fat ourselves we are put at further risk, unless we consume exclusively organically farmed produce, meats, and dairy products.

Breast milk can carry over two hundred chemical pollutants because it is so high in fat. It is estimated that, during breastfeeding, babies are exposed to a level of environmental toxins forty times higher than at any time later in their life. However, even with this contamination, we must continue to breastfeed our babies, for the immunological benefits of mother's milk still far outweigh this relatively high-level exposure.

Foods and Cooking Methods That Increase the Risk of Cancer

Foods. Looking more specifically at the elements within the diet that produce cancer, it is clear that excessive meat and animal fats put us at greater risk. While a high intake of red meat appears to increase the risk of colorectal cancer, the roles of other protein foods such as fish, chicken, and dairy products are unclear. In case-control studies, a high intake of dietary fat has been associated with increased risk of many cancers, including breast, prostate, lung, and colorectal. This association, however, has not been confirmed consistently in research. It has not been possible so far to distinguish between the effects of total, saturated, vegetable, and animal fats. The inconsistencies in these findings may reflect varying biological effects of different fatty acids such as the omega-3 or omega-6 fatty acids, some of which may be beneficial and some adverse for tumor growth.

Links Between Specific Cancers and Dietary Factors

Cancer Site	Adverse Dietary Factors
Breast	Total fat, omega-6 fatty acids, meat, alcohol
Colon and rectum	Total fat, meat, heterocyclic amines, alcohol (especially beer)
Stomach	Nitrates/nitrites, alcohol, salted and smoked foods
Esophagus	Alcohol
Endometrium and ovaries	Saturated fat
Prostate	Saturated fat
Pancreas	Coffee
Bladder	Coffee
Lung	Saturated fat, meat

Cooking Methods. There is evidence that charbroiling meat and fats, and superheating fats, create dangerous free radicals and carcinogenic compounds such as polycyclic aromatic hydrocarbons. For the same reason, there is concern about the safety of smoked foods. Excessively salted and pickled foods also increase the risk of cancer, as do those that are preserved with saltpeter (potassium nitrate), such as salamis. A direct link has been identified between salted fish consumed in south China and a type of cancer found in the nose or throat area. There is also an increased incidence of gastric cancer in the Far East, where higher levels of salt and salt-preserved foods are eaten.

Another very specific food contaminant that is definitely implicated in liver cancer in undeveloped countries is aflatoxin, a metabolic product of a fungus that contaminates grains stored in hot and humid conditions.

Protective Factors in Food

Fortunately, it is not all bad news. People who eat large amounts of fruits and vegetables cut their cancer risk in half. The most consistent observation is a decrease in cancers of the lung, stomach, and esophagus, and a smaller but consistent decrease in cancers of the mouth, larynx, colon, breast, pancreas, and bladder. Strangely, the same protection has not been seen in cancer of the prostate.

Cancers protected against most strongly by a healthy diet are those of the mouth, pharynx (throat), larynx (voice box), stomach, colon (large intestine), and rectum. The next most protected against are cancers of the breast, lung, prostate, endometrium (uterine lining), and ovaries.

Initially, investigations into fruit and vegetables centered around the protective effects of antioxidant vitamins, particularly beta-carotene and vitamin E, and the effects of fiber. Studies were initiated after scientists discovered that blood levels of beta-carotene were higher in people who ate large amounts of fruit and vegetables, and that these people also enjoyed lower cancer incidence and suffered fewer deaths from cancer. This led to the hypothesis that the beta-carotene itself conveyed the protection.

However, subsequent research in which individuals were given beta-carotene in tablet form to try to prevent cancer has proved very confusing. In some studies, smokers who took beta-carotene ended up having a higher cancer risk than those who did not! Critics say these results are invalid because synthetic rather than natural beta-carotene was used.

Overall, the research showed that people with high levels of beta-carotene in their bloodstream at the beginning of the trial were better protected than those with low levels. It was those whose levels increased very rapidly during the course of the trial who seemed to be at increased risk of lung cancer. From this evidence, we can deduce that beta-carotene alone does not convey the benefit; work is now underway to investigate the contribution of the many families of plant chemicals (phytochemicals) that are thought to be implicated in cancer prevention.

Studies on the role of vitamin E are more promising. Results showed that 50 milligrams per day of vitamin E reduced the risk of prostate cancer by 40 percent. It is also thought that calcium, vitamin D, and folic acid may all reduce the risk of cancers of the colon and rectum. Other studies highlight the role of the antioxidant vitamins C, E, and beta-carotene, and the mineral selenium in helping to prevent colon polyps from turning malignant.

The most exciting work in the last decade was done with the phytochemicals in green leafy vegetables and broccoli, in yellow and orange vegetables such as yellow peppers and carrots, and in onions, tomatoes, and soy products. Cabbages and broccoli (and other brassicas) were found to contain a compound called *indoleglycosinate*, which protects against cancer. The yellow and orange vegetables were found to contain a combination of factors, including many carotenoids, calcium, selenium, and other micronutrients that work in concert to produce a strong anticancer effect. Tomatoes contain a substance called *lycopene*, and studies show an inverse relationship between bodily lycopene levels and cancers of the digestive tract and prostate. Soy products and fermented soy products such as miso contain phytoestrogens, which block estrogen activity in the same way as the anticancer drug tamoxifen. The plant chemicals—phytates, protease inhibitors, lignins, isoflavonoids, and isoflavones—are under investigation too, as they are all thought to be direct inhibitors of cancer genes. Studies with miso—fermented soy or barley—show that it offers definite cancer-protective effects. Lemons have been shown to contain another anticancer substance, called *limonene*.

Other anticancer agents, which interfere with both initiation and promotion of cancer cells, have been found in shiitake mushrooms, kombu, and kelp. Phytochemicals from fruits and vegetables that are believed to help protect against cancer include plant phenols, aromatic isothiocyanates, thiocyanates, methylated flavones, coumarins, saponins, allium compounds, plant sterols, dithiolthiones, glucosinates, and indoles, as well as naturally occurring plant selenium, zinc, copper, iron, calcium, manganese, potassium, and magnesium salts (see Appendix 5 for a full list). Naturally occurring ascorbic acid (vitamin C) and its accompanying bioflavonoids and cofactors (now thought to be as important as the vitamin itself), tocopherols, B vitamins (including folic acid, B6, and riboflavin), retinols, and carotenoids are also very important elements of fruit and vegetables that protect us from cancer. Many of these work together symbiotically to render carcinogenic substances harmless and to repair damage to DNA in a cell's nucleus, thereby preventing tumor formation.

Protease inhibitors, like those found in soy, are thought to protect cells from ionizing radioactivity from natural sources as well as from X rays used in cancer therapy and diagnostic procedures.

Plant constituents such as the flavonoids and plant estrogens have been shown, in small studies, to alter the blood levels of sex hormones associated with prostate and breast cancer risk, but direct links have yet to be demonstrated. However, the ability to demonstrate a biological basis for diet/cancer associations in population studies considerably strengthens confidence that these relationships are causal. It is thought, for example, that the high levels of phytoestrogens in soy products give protection from breast cancer to women in Japan, where the lifetime risk is only one in forty-five, compared with one in ten in the West.

Fiber in the diet is thought to protect us in two ways. First, the phytates and lignins in fiber directly lower the production of free radicals within the body. High fiber levels in the diet also speed up the transit time of potential carcinogens through the intestine, thereby decreasing their absorption rate and lessening the harmful effect on the gut tissues they come in contact with. It is therefore likely that a healthy, whole-food (that is, emphasizing foods close to their original, natural form rather than processed foods), predominantly vegetarian diet protects against cancer by providing adequate levels of vitamins, minerals, and phytochemicals in order to:

❖ promote healthy tissue growth and replication

❖ boost immune function

❖ deactivate dangerous free radicals and pollutants

❖ directly stabilize cell membranes and cell-division processes

❖ promote DNA and RNA repair and proto-oncogene stabilization

It appears that our grandmothers were right when they told us, "Vegetables are good for you"—and not just for skin and hair! It is absolutely vital that we pay proper attention to diet, both as individuals and in society. We must all adopt a healthy diet—not only in our homes, but also in our restaurants, schools, hospitals, and all other institutions—if we are even to begin the fight and win the war against cancer.

Smoking
Smoking causes 30 percent of cancer deaths.

Current knowledge implicates smoking in no fewer than fourteen different cancers. Compared with nonsmokers, cigarette smokers are:

❖ 15 times more likely to have lung cancer

❖ 10 times more likely to have cancer of the larynx (voice box) or pharynx (throat)

❖ 7 times more likely to have cancer of the esophagus (gullet)

❖ 4 times more likely to have cancer of the pelvis, kidney, or mouth

❖ 3 times more likely to have cancer of the bladder

❖ 2 times more likely to have cancer of the pancreas

❖ 1.5 times more likely to have cancer of the lip, nose, stomach, kidney, and liver, and myeloid leukemia

Pipe and cigar smoking are also important contributing factors in cancers of the mouth, pharynx (throat), esophagus (gullet), and larynx (voice box), and pipe smoking is also linked to cancer of the lip. The risk of many of these cancers—especially liver cancers—is further compounded by alcohol consumption. In 1995, Sir Richard Peto and Sir Richard Doll estimated that in developed countries smoking was responsible for 39 percent of all cancer deaths in men

Percentage of Deaths from Cancer Attributable to Smoking (in 1995)

Country	% Male	% Female
Australia	32	14
Denmark	38	22
France	38	2
Hungary	53	15
Italy	42	6
Japan	29	8
Netherlands	45	9
Russian Federation	55	6
Spain	34	0
Sweden	20	8
UK	40	20
United States	45	28

(Permission to reprint granted by Sir Richard Doll.)

and 15 percent in women. Sadly, the figure for women continues to increase as more women start to smoke. There is considerable variation in the male/female ratios throughout the developed countries of the world.

Smoking-related cancer deaths have generally increased over the last twenty years. Among men in France they have risen from 33 to 38 percent. But in some countries they have decreased, most notably in the UK, where they have dropped from 52 percent to 40 percent among men. In women, however, the proportions have all increased, except in Spain, where they are still immeasurably low because few women have been smoking for long enough for any substantial effect to be detected.

It has been shown beyond doubt that half of all regular smokers die prematurely from a smoking-related disease. As well as causing cancer, smoking is an important cause of heart attacks, strokes, chronic lung conditions, and circulation problems that can result in pain, gangrene, and leg amputation. Smoking also causes tooth and gum problems and is a significant cause of peptic ulcers.

Despite the very well publicized dangers of cigarette smoking, roughly one in four adults in Western countries over the age of eighteen still smokes. A recent alarming trend is that tobacco companies have begun to transfer their marketing efforts to developing countries, as advertising restrictions become tighter and tighter in the West. This will result in the most dire consequences and suffering, since most developing countries cannot even provide morphine for palliative care for people with cancer, let alone screening, medical treatment, and hospice care.

The reason for the terrible medical consequences of smoking is that cigarette smoke is estimated to contain some forty different carcinogenic and irritant chemicals. In addition, the heat of the cigarette smoke and the cigarette end (especially in unfiltered cigarettes) can cause direct burning and irritation to the lips, throat, and windpipe. This continual burning irritation can create ideal conditions for cancer to develop. Attempts to lower one's risk by smoking low-tar cigarettes have backfired in many cases, because smokers of low-tar cigarettes often inhale more deeply to get the same levels of nicotine. As a result, different patterns of lung cancer are now being seen, with the tumor situated far deeper in the lung tissue.

People continue to smoke because nicotine and other chemicals in cigarette smoke are highly addictive, and the chemical "buzz" smoking creates gives them temporary relief from tension and anxiety. Many people use cigarettes as a social and psychological prop to help them deal with constant anxiety and stress. To kick the habit, people often need emotional support to deal with these feelings.

Reproductive Hormones
Excess hormones cause 10 percent of cancer deaths.

The problem with reproductive hormones occurs when we are exposed to an excess of hormones to which we are not evolutionarily adjusted. As was mentioned in the section on dietary causes of cancer, both an excess of calories (and the obesity this causes) and the consumption of animal fats lead to unhealthily high hormone levels within the body. This means that throughout our lifetimes, our bodies undergo much higher circulating levels of these hormones than our ancestors' bodies did.

In developing countries, where people have a far lower nutritional intake than is now common in developed countries, girls start their menstrual cycle later and women have multiple pregnancies followed by prolonged lactation. All three of these factors greatly reduce the risks of cancer of the breast, endometrium, and ovaries. Later menstruation and the hormones associated with pregnancy and lactation reduce estrogen activity in the body. Estrogen is a very powerful hormone that prepares the lining of the uterus for conception, the egg for release from the ovary, and the breast for the possibility of conception and subsequent lactation. In women who repeatedly go through the menstrual cycle without conceiving, the monthly estrogenic stimulation of the tissues can lead to cancer development. If background levels of estrogen in the body are already high due to obesity and diet, the problem is compounded.

Added to this problem is the additional use of estrogen hormones in birth control pills and hormone replacement therapy (HRT), both of which have been shown to increase the risk of cancer. The Pill and HRT increase the risk of breast cancer during the period they are actually being taken, and even the Combined Pill, which contains estrogen and progesterone, increases the risk of breast cancer by 20 percent. However, with the Pill this risk disappears once a woman stops taking it. At the same time, the Pill protects against cancer of the endometrium (uterine lining) and ovaries by up to 50 percent in the long term—and protection continues even after the woman has stopped taking it. Medical authorities argue that because the breast cancer rate is much lower in young women than in postmenopausal women, the risk of taking the Pill while young is acceptable and is outweighed by the future protection of the endometrium and ovaries.

With HRT, the increased risk of breast and endometrial cancer after ten to twenty-five years on the treatment is estimated at 20 percent, and the risk remains the same five years after stopping. But it has also been shown that taking HRT reduces the risk of colon cancer by around 20 percent.

As you can see, the hormone picture is complicated, and we in the West are certainly not about to revert to a lifestyle in which women have multiple pregnancies! The medical answer has been to suggest that women be given a synthetic estrogen hormone blockade to protect them from high estrogen levels, and therefore from breast cancer, by use of the drug tamoxifen. In fact, a huge trial currently is being conducted to look at the possibility of using tamoxifen on a widespread basis to help reduce breast cancer incidence and mortality. This has become a main plank of the research strategy for the big cancer-research organizations, but it is a path strongly opposed by many women's action groups, which feel that the side effects of tamoxifen are being grossly underplayed. The most notable concern is the increased risk by 5–10 percent of endometrial (uterine-lining) cancer while taking tamoxifen. The medical charities' response to this is to say that tamoxifen's protection against breast cancer is fifty times greater than its risk to the uterine lining, and that the benefits therefore outweigh the side effects.

However, other serious side effects of tamoxifen can include severe weight gain; diarrhea; nausea; and skin, hair, and even voice changes. As we know, obesity is a risk factor for breast cancer, and so taking tamoxifen can create a vicious cycle. In my view, it would seem far more appropriate for us to tackle the problem of obesity and excessive fat consumption, rather than taking this "chemo-preventive" route with all its associated dangers. The next chapter will give clear advice for women facing these hormonal dilemmas.

The medical profession offers no equivalent solution for the prevention of cancer of the prostate, apart from the possible benefits of taking vitamin E. It is believed, however, that ultimately cancer of the testis will be preventable by a change in some lifestyle or environmental factor; the fact that its incidence increased so dramatically in the latter half of the last century indicates that something we are doing differently must be causing the problem.

Infection
Infection causes 10 percent of cancer deaths.

A large number of cancers worldwide are caused by parasites, bacteria, and viruses, and it is likely that as our understanding increases, the assessment of the percentage risk from these agents to the cause of cancer will grow. The role of bacteria and parasites is much greater in developing countries, whereas the role of viruses is more ubiquitous. In Africa and Asia, many cancers of the bladder, colon (large intestine), liver, and bile ducts are caused by parasite infections, all of which could be avoided with a combination of environmental and therapeutic measures. These parasites play little or no role in cancer causation in developed countries.

The role of bacteria in causing cancer of the stomach and digestive tract has received much attention recently, while the role of bacteria in cancer of the large intestine has been questioned. Until recently, the theory was that gut bacteria may turn bile salts into carcinogens, but at present this theory looks less likely. On the other hand, the recently discovered *Helicobacter pylori* bacterium has been shown to significantly contribute to cancer of the stomach, as well as to stomach ulcers. This is not a straightforward relationship, however, because in other countries where the incidence of *Helicobacter* is high, there is a low incidence of cancer of the stomach. Even more confusing is the finding that where *Helicobacter* is eradicated through antibiotics used to treat gastric ulcers, the incidence of esophageal and lung cancer increases!

It is possible that chronic bacterial infection of the bladder may be a cause of bladder cancer, because the bacteria can produce waste products (called *nitrosamines*) that are carcinogenic and over time may cause the disease.

Viral Causes of Cancer

Virus	Cancer
Hepatitis B	Hepatocarcinoma
Hepatitis C	Hepatocarcinoma
Human papillomavirus (HPV), types 16, 18, and others	Cancer of the cervix, vulva, vagina, penis, and anus
Human herpes type 4 (Epstein-Barr virus)	Lymphoma, immunoblastic lymphoma, nasal T-cell lymphoma, Hodgkin's disease, nasopharyngeal cancer
Human herpes type 8	Kaposi's sarcoma
Kaposi's associated herpes virus	Body-cavity lymphoma
Human T-cell leukemia type 1	Adult T-cell leukemia/lymphoma
Simian virus 40-like	Ependymoma, choroid plexus tumors, mesothelioma, and bone tumors
Herpes simplex type 2 (genital herpes)	Cancer of the vagina, penis, and anus
Human immunodeficiency virus (HIV)	Lymphoma
Acquired immune deficiency syndrome (AIDS)	Kaposi's sarcoma

(Permission to reprint granted by Sir Richard Doll.)

Viruses are a much bigger and more serious cause of cancer altogether, responsible for the great majority of two of the most common cancers worldwide: of the liver and of the cervix. They are also involved in many of the less common cancers. Strangely, the viruses listed below are not associated with every case of the cancers they can cause. Also, it is often found that compounding factors need to be involved before the viruses cause a problem. For example, the virus that causes Burkitt's lymphoma in Africa has its effect in the presence of malarial parasites, and in many cases the virus causing liver cancer has its effect in the presence of aflatoxin. HPV, HIV, and the herpes viruses can all be transmitted sexually (as can hepatitis C on rare occasions). The practice of safe sex has therefore far wider importance than the public currently realizes. We have been given a very strong message about safe sex in relation to HIV, but the message is much less strong in relation to HPV, which is a significant cause of cervical cancer and premature death in women.

The medical profession is concentrating its efforts on the role of vaccinations in preventing these virally triggered cancers. It is already possible to immunize against hepatitis, and widespread immunization is being introduced in some tropical and semitropical countries where hepatitis infection is more common than in developed countries. It is hoped that the HPV vaccine will be available to women within ten years, in particular to help prevent cervical cancer.

It is certainly my hunch that viruses set the scene for many more of the common cancers than we currently realize. Viruses transmitted through the animal food chain may yet turn out to be the real reason why the eating of meat and other animal products is so strongly implicated in increased cancer risk.

Alcohol

Alcohol causes 5 percent of cancer deaths.

Alcohol is estimated to cause an average of 5 percent of cancer deaths in developed countries, but the rates can vary from 3 percent to as much as 12 percent in different countries. Heavy drinkers are:

- ❖ 3 times more likely to have cancer of the esophagus (gullet) than nondrinkers
- ❖ 2 times more likely to have cancers of the mouth, pharynx (throat), and larynx (voice box)
- ❖ 1.5 times more likely to have cancer of the liver
- ❖ 1.2 times more likely to have breast cancer

The role of alcohol in the development of breast cancer is the most recent discovery of all these associations. It is thought that this effect is caused by alcohol's ability to raise hormone levels in the body. Evidence gathered in 1993 by investigators at Reichmann research laboratories (showing that alcohol increased the level of estrogens in the blood) put the causal relationship between alcohol and breast cancer beyond reasonable doubt. The risks were assessed on the basis of an "average consumption" of alcohol. The risk increases in heavy drinkers. The high-risk levels associated with cancers of the mouth, throat, gullet, and voice box are all significantly lower in nonsmokers who drink heavily.

The message for us all is to reduce our drinking dramatically— you can still have a glass of wine or beer, but stick within the safe limits of two units a day for women, three for men. Indeed, other evidence shows that a small amount of alcohol (one glass of wine per day) can reduce the risk of heart attack. Some people argue that this is a good reason to continue a low level of alcohol consumption. However, it is likely that the cardiovascular protection is caused by the relaxing effect of alcohol and the nutritional benefits of the vitamins and minerals in wine. These effects can easily be achieved in safer ways, through self-help practices such as yoga, meditation, relaxation, and a healthy diet, without any of alcohol's toxicity to the body, so don't feel you have to drink to stay healthy.

Anyone who has ever drunk too much or suffered a hangover can be under no illusion whatsoever about the toxicity of alcohol. Its role in degenerative disease of many kinds has been proved beyond any shadow of doubt. The liver, gut, mental health, social, and cancer problems created by alcohol make it public enemy number two after smoking. If alcohol were introduced now as a new drug, it would probably be judged a Class A illegal substance because of the profound risks associated with its use. Unfortunately, alcohol use is so deeply embedded within Western culture as our major recreational drug that any governmental attempt to control its consumption would probably result in civil war! So once again, it comes down to the role of the individual in changing behavior patterns if there is to be any improvement in alcohol-related cancer statistics.

For many people, changing their use of alcohol represents an even more serious challenge than giving up smoking; addressing this challenge will be given serious consideration in the next chapter. Certainly, of the two, the priority is to give up smoking, because this will at least reduce the risk of lung cancer as well as decrease the risk to the windpipe and gullet posed by alcohol.

Electromagnetic Radiation
EMR causes 4 percent of cancer deaths.

In developed countries, ultraviolet radiation from sunlight is responsible for most melanomas and nearly all squamous and basal-cell cancers of the skin. Added to this is the effect of naturally occurring radioactivity or background radioactivity, which is produced naturally by radon and its decay products in the earth.

Radioactivity

Naturally occurring radioactivity is linked to the presence of radon gas. The U.S. surgeon general has warned that radon is the second leading cause of lung cancer in the United States today. Only smoking causes more lung cancer deaths. The effects of radon and smoking act synergistically; thus stopping smoking makes radon exposure far less dangerous. As far as natural sources of radioactivity go, it is possible to ascertain the radon levels in your area from state environmental agencies; and, if you are concerned, your home can be checked for radon gas (see the Resources section). In fact, the U.S. Environmental Protection Agency and the surgeon general recommend that all homes below the third floor and all schools be checked for radon.

There is also widespread concern about the effects of radioactive leakage and contamination from nuclear power stations and nuclear waste dumping. Controversy continues about the role of nuclear power stations in cancer causation, but certainly clusters of childhood leukemia have been seen around power stations. It is possible that power-station workers and local people are being affected by radioactive contamination, and that these effects are being passed on to their offspring through affected sperm or eggs.

The ethics of nuclear power remain, in my opinion, highly questionable. It seems irresponsible to create more and more radioactive material and waste material that as yet cannot be eliminated and that has to buried or dumped in the sea where it will remain radioactive for extremely long periods. To leave this ghastly legacy for future generations over thousands of years to come is an appalling crime against humanity and nature, and it seems very wrong that it is legal to do so.

Nuclear accidents and exposure to radioactive materials of any sort are associated with very marked increases in cancer incidence. After the Chernobyl disaster, levels of thyroid cancer in the region rose dramatically due to the spillage of radioactive iodine that then became concentrated in the thyroid glands of people living within a considerable radius of the site. The main cause of death in those who are not killed outright by a nuclear explosion is cancer, which can continue appearing for years after the original blast.

Medical X rays are also a source of considerable concern. It has been shown that X rays to the mother's abdomen during pregnancy cause 5 percent of leukemias in children.

Individually, we must take the utmost care to ensure that, if possible, we are not living or working close to sources of radiation—either natural radioactivity from the earth in the form of radon, or the manmade variety in military weapons, chemical factories, power stations, or nuclear dumps. People who work or live near sources of radiation must remain vigilant and keep in close touch with local authorities for constant information and reassurance about levels of radioactivity in the area and the proper implementation of safety measures.

Unproven, but of concern, is the effect of radiation emitted from computer screens on our brains and immune systems. There is some evidence of increased incidence of brain tumors, leukemias, and lymphomas in those who sit in front of computers day after day. The general advice for people who spend long hours in front of a computer is to use a screen to help defuse the radiation emitted and to take regular breaks.

Ultraviolet Radiation

Atmospheric pollution has played a serious role in increasing our risk of skin cancer. The three main skin cancers—melanoma, squamous-cell cancer, and basal-cell cancer—are all caused by overexposure to UV light. Normally, the ozone layer mops up the majority of ultraviolet light from the sun. But because of the damage to the ozone layer and the resulting hole that has been created by CFCs from refrigerators and aerosol cans, people are being exposed to far higher levels of ultraviolet radiation than normal. Certainly this has had an adverse effect on skin cancer incidence in Australia, which has been particularly badly affected.

Ultraviolet light is made up of UVA, UVB, and UVC rays. Usually, only a small amount of UVA and UVB reaches the earth. It is the UVB rays that burn our skin and that are probably the most important cancer-producing agent. But in recent years, experimental studies in animals have suggested that UVA rays penetrate the skin layer more deeply than UVB rays (without burning it) and may also play an important role in cancer development. Individuals with pale skin or freckles, blue eyes, red or fair hair and who burn easily in the sun are more prone to skin damage than those with olive or dark skins, and should be particularly careful.

It is also important to remember that UVA rays from suntanning beds can potentially overstimulate our skin. The beds have been declared safe by medical authorities, but as with so many things, it is all a matter of degree. There is also the question of whether the machine is working according to the manufacturer's specifications.

Cancer researchers go as far as saying that there is no such thing as a healthy tan. Their advice is to avoid getting a suntan altogether and to wear sunblock and protective clothing when in hot countries. If a tanned look is desired, their advice would be to avoid the use of tanning beds and to opt instead for tanning lotions, which stain the skin.

Electricity

Another source of concern is the possible link between cancer and electromagnetic radiation from electrical power lines, electrical towers, high-voltage units, and electrical household equipment. Recently, a correlation has been found between extra-low-frequency electric fields and the incidence of childhood leukemia and male breast cancer. There is also an observed risk of brain tumors in electric-company workers.

In the past, it has been hard to prove any connection between the electromagnetic fields (EMF) of high-voltage electrical equipment and cancer. But recent work in Bristol shows that in some situations it may not be the electromagnetic field itself that is creating a hazard, but radioactive particles that are attracted into the field. It is unwise to live and work close to high-voltage electrical equipment of any sort or to live over buried electrical cabling.

In general, our environments are becoming more and more electrical, and it is not unusual to work in buildings with many hundreds of computer terminals surrounded by layer upon layer of electrical cabling within the walls. If you are concerned, contact your local electric utility; some will test for EMF levels in homes and businesses. Otherwise, it may be possible to find a private environmental-testing lab that will test for EMF levels.

Radio Waves and Microwaves

In addition to being surrounded by electrical fields, we are being bombarded by radio waves and microwaves from ever increasing broadcasting and the rapidly rising use of mobile phones. There is much concern about the microwave emanations from mobile phones themselves and their possible link with brain cancer. Currently, medical authorities feel the risk is small, but the picture is still far from clear.

Questions also exist about the effects of the many radio and telephone towers being erected throughout cities and the country-side and the role of radio waves and microwaves on our genetic material. It is clear that, once again, the commercial sector is racing ahead of the scientists and that the telecommunications industry has not yet fully researched the potential risks of the equipment it is installing and selling.

Microwave ovens are another source of potential risk if they are used improperly or if they are faulty and directly expose the user to microwaves. Microwaved food may itself cause trauma to the mouth, esophagus (gullet), and stomach if proper cooling times are not observed. Microwave energy is a very high-frequency energy, which heats food rapidly to temperatures beyond those reached by normal cooking methods. While this is questionable nutritionally—because vitamins and vital plant enzymes and phytochemicals are destroyed at high temperatures—it is also probable that if the intense microwave radiation is not allowed to dissipate properly before the food is eaten, it can cause burning and tissue damage to the digestive tract. Repeated irritation to the mucus membrane in this way could easily be a cause of future cancer.

Clearly, there is still a great deal we do not know about microwave technology, and until the science is clearer, great care should be taken in the use of mobile phones and microwave ovens.

Sound

Another little-researched and little-understood subject is the effect of sound on the body. At certain frequencies sound can have both very beneficial and very damaging effects on human tissue. There is some concern about the use of ultrasound in medical practice and whether this is a cause of cancer. I also question the effect of sound in dance clubs, where young people are bombarded with increasingly loud and chaotic noise. Some clubs even place speakers under the floor as well as on the walls in order to send intense vibrational energy through the feet of the dancers while they are listening to the music, though the vibrations they feel through the floor are slightly out of phase with what they are hearing. Again, these practices are being employed without any knowledge as to the potential damage created by subjecting the body to these intense, chaotic vibrational patterns.

Earth Energies

More controversial is the question of the earth's electromagnetic field and the role of the currents created by the underlying rock formation. The "earth energies" and "lay lines" created have been implicated in the development of cancer. Studies by dowsers who can track these currents show very specific clusters of cancer along the lay lines in cities that have been fully mapped. This is an area that as yet has received no serious scientific study, but it is one that should be looked into by individuals and cancer researchers, for the correlations are too high to be ignored. It may well be that a strange underlying phenomenon like this will solve the mystery of the often seemingly random nature of cancer distribution among people who are all broadly exposed to the same risk factors.

Environmental Pollution

Pollution causes 2 percent of cancer deaths.

Public concern about environmental pollution and cancer is very high, although medical authorities estimate that it causes only 2 percent of cancer deaths. The main areas of concern are:

❖ industrial waste

❖ pollution of the air with diesel and gasoline fumes and the products of waste (particularly plastic) combustion

❖ by-products of intensive agriculture

❖ chemicals used at home, in food additives, and in building, cleaning, and gardening products

Asbestos

Asbestos, which was used extensively in building during the twentieth century for roofing, insulation, and as part of floor tiles, is one very specific substance that has been proved beyond doubt to be associated with cancer of the lining of the lung (mesothelioma). Asbestos fibers crumble easily, releasing microscopic particles into the air. These are inhaled deeply into the lung tissue or swallowed; they can lodge in the throat and lungs, and sometimes travel into the gut, causing damage in the stomach and intestine, in some cases leading to cancer. In addition to causing mesothelioma, asbestos has been implicated in cancer of the larynx (voice box) and also possibly of the esophagus (gullet), stomach, and ovaries. The worst kinds of asbestos are the blue and brown varieties. The white kind is less dangerous because the body is more able to eliminate it.

Very strict guidelines now exist for the use and removal of asbestos from buildings, and it is most unwise for untrained individuals to deal with any asbestos problem in the home, whatever type of asbestos is involved. If there is any concern about the presence of asbestos—for example, it may have become damaged through age—it is vital to obtain the help of experts who are certified by the local environmental agencies to advise on its removal.

Persistent Chemicals

Great concern has developed about the effect of industrial, transportation, waste disposal, and farming pollution because of the dangerous persistent chemicals these practices leave in the environment. Environmentalists have reported cancers in fish linked to the pollution of lakes with polycyclic aromatic hydrocarbons found in petroleum products, and mass sterility among wildlife. This, combined with falling sperm levels in human males, has triggered widespread anxiety about the cancer risk to humans from environmental carcinogens and about tumor promotion by hormonally active pollutants known as *endocrine disrupters*.

A Danish study found that the average sperm count dropped by 45 percent between 1940 and 1990. The volume of the semen ejaculated had also dropped by 25 percent, making an effective sperm decline of 50 percent. There was also a big increase in the rates of testicular cancer among young men during the same period. Exposure of male babies in the womb to elevated estrogen levels (from diet and chemical estrogens in the environment) may increase the risk of testicular tumors, prostate cancer, and benign prostatic disease in later life.

Environmental campaigners have homed in on the possible role of hormone-mimicking organochlorine pesticides in the development of cancer. Past and current use of organochlorine pesticides has led to pollution of the entire globe, with detectable levels in the body fat of nearly everyone worldwide. Of particular concern is the question of whether organochlorine pesticides are one of the environmental factors responsible for the rise in breast cancer, because of their estrogen-mimicking activity. The persistence of these chemicals in the environment, and their accumulation in animals at the top of the food chain, has led to the introduction of measures to control their use. In the United States many organochlorine pesticides—including DDT, aldrin, and dieldrin—have been banned, and certain others are classified as "severely restricted." However, DDT and other organochlorine pesticides are still widely used in many parts of the world, although the United Nations has established a voluntary "right-to-know" procedure to inform importing countries of potential hazards with these substances.

Packaging, particularly plastic, is another source of hormone-disrupting chemicals. They may also be found in ointments, cosmetics, shampoos, and other common household products. A large number of manmade chemicals (as well as a few natural ones) that have been released into the environment have the potential to disrupt the hormone systems of animals, including humans. Among these are the persistent, bioaccumulative organohalogen compounds found in some pesticides, fungicides, herbicides, insecticides, industrial chemicals, other synthetic products, and some metals.

Examples of chemicals in the environment known to disrupt the endocrine system are listed in Appendix 1. If they find their way into the body, many of these compounds imitate the action of estrogen. Unless the environmental load of synthetic hormone or endocrine disrupters is abated and controlled, large-scale problems in the population are possible. In studies on rats, organochlorine compounds have been shown to aggravate already existing breast tumors, although none of the pesticides actually triggered the breast cancer. The argument against these chemicals is weakened, however, by the fact that, in reality, most people have been exposed to fairly minuscule amounts of organochlorine pesticides through food, and in the UK, for one, levels in body tissues are low and have been falling.

Several studies have compared pesticide levels in women with breast cancer to levels in women without the disease. In a New York study, women with the highest blood levels of DDE (a breakdown product of DDT) were four times more likely to develop breast cancer than women with the lowest levels. Similar but insignificant trends were found in three other case-controlled studies. However, in a much larger study of three hundred women—half of whom had breast cancer—there was no significant relation between DDE levels and the disease. Taking all the research and arguments into account, the evidence that organochlorine pesticides increase the risk of breast cancer is fairly weak. However, we must continue to strive vigorously toward organic farming for many other ecological and health reasons, most particularly to raise the nutritional quality of our food.

Agricultural Practices

Another source of potential pollution are agricultural processes that contribute to nitrate contamination of food and water. These include the plowing up of grassland for arable farming (the grass leaks nitrates into the soil), the excessive use of mineral fertilizers, poor management of slurry from animal husbandry, and inappropriate use of organic fertilizer. The problem arises when nitrates are converted to nitrosamines in the body; most nitrosamines that have been tested are carcinogenic in animals. Within the body, the antioxidant vitamins C and E prevent nitrosamines from forming.

Certain types of vegetables, such as spinach and lettuce, are nitrophilic—that is, they accumulate more nitrates from the soil than they can convert into protein. Organically grown nitrophilic vegetables are less contaminated with nitrates than conventional vegetables. This is another argument for choosing organic vegetables.

However, because increased vegetable consumption provides the body with a rich source of antioxidants, the net effect is that high vegetable consumption protects against digestive tract cancers regardless of the presence of nitrates in the vegetables and the presence of pesticides and fertilizers. There is no real support from studies that nitrates in vegetables cause cancer, and there are inconsistent results demonstrating an association between cancer and nitrates in drinking water. And so, again, evidence about the possible role of nitrates in the development of cancer is weak and conflicting.

Another area of concern within intensive farming is the use of growth promoters—a mixed bag of hormones, antibiotics, beta-agonists, and copper, among others—in animal husbandry to increase milk and meat production. Of these, the one chemical that could be potentially linked to cancer is growth hormone. The United States is virtually the only Western nation that does not ban the use of genetically engineered Bovine Growth Hormone (rBGH); both Canada and the European Union ban it. In addition to agitating the U.S. Food and Drug Administration (FDA) or the appropriate congressional representatives to change this regulation and ban the use of rBGH, concerned citizens of the world should work to ensure that the use of growth hormones is not adopted in developing countries.

With regard to the use of antibiotics and copper as feed additives, although many other health concerns exist, there is no obvious mechanism by which these substances could contribute to cancer.

Conventional wisdom suggests that animal hormones in the meat and dairy products we eat do not produce biological activity in the human body. However, once again it may be a matter of degree. For people with a diet heavily oriented toward animal foods, with high levels of butter, cream, cheese, milk, and meat, the intake of animal hormones may compound the hormone-raising effects of obesity potentially caused by this type of diet.

Genetic Modification

The possible relationship between the production of genetically modified crops and future cancer is a very topical issue. The subject of genetic modification is an emotionally charged subject, because changing genetic material is the starting point of the whole cancer process. Even with the natural, built-in levels of protection against genetic mutation within the body, our genetic material is highly vulnerable in today's world, as the soaring rates of cancer show. To introduce another element of disruption into the genetic blueprint of nature would seem, potentially, to be pouring fuel on the fire, inviting genetic catastrophe in the future.

It is always reckless to introduce significant scientific or technological change before the repercussions are fully understood. In the realms of both genetics and technology, we are seeing development that is far outstripping our ability to foresee where this evolutionary path will take us, let alone the profound consequences it may have for nature and humankind. I therefore feel that if we wish to protect ourselves from cancer over the long term, we should be extremely cautious about genetic modification and stick to working with nature rather than trying to modify it.

Regulation and Taking Action

Even though the cancer threat from environmental pollution is currently thought to be relatively small, we must avoid being complacent. The environmental situation may well have a bearing on the cancer risk associated with food and infection, and certainly the effects of sunlight are worsened by the results of pollution on the ozone layer. The situation is worsening as traffic pollution increases, and as hundreds, possibly thousands, of new synthetic chemicals go on the market each year, faster than toxicologists and regulatory agencies are able to develop new ways to detect and check them. As Theo Colburn writes in her impressive book *Our Stolen Future*, an investigation into the effect of industrial pollution on wildlife and human health:

> What is happening to the animals in Florida, English rivers, the Baltic, the High Arctic, the Great Lakes and Lake Baikal in Siberia has immediate relevance to humans. The damage seen in wildlife has ominously foreshadowed symptoms that appear to be increasing in the human population. Humans and animals share the common environment as well as the common genetic evolutionary legacy. Living in a man-made landscape we easily forget that our well-being is rooted in natural systems yet all human enterprise rests on the foundation of natural systems, that provide a myriad of invisible life support services. Our connections to these natural systems may be less direct and obvious than those of an eagle or an otter but we are no less deeply implicated in life's web.

While the contribution of environmental pollution to cancer appears small, a great deal is still unknown and constant vigilance is necessary. It is absolutely crucial that we all develop a sense of the sacredness of our environment, and take action to protect it both by doing our bit at home and by setting up green initiatives in our places of work and communities. It is imperative that anyone wishing to prevent cancer, personally or collectively, become involved in and actively support environmental organizations and continue to lobby local lawmakers and all political parties to ensure that they keep the protection of the environment at the very top of their agenda.

Household Carcinogens

Because our homes are where we spend the majority of our time, it is particularly important to think about our exposure to cancer-causing chemicals (carcinogens) there.

The main risks in the home are:

❖ secondhand smoke (the intake of cigarette, pipe, or tobacco smoke from other family members, or guests, who smoke)

❖ chemicals found in cleaners, solvents, pesticides, and cosmetics, and in products used in home-repair projects, decorating, and hobbies

Increasingly, the potential risk of cancer from household products and cosmetics whose use we take for granted is being brought to our attention. Household products that can contain carcinogens include:

Disinfectants, all-purpose cleaners, bathroom cleaner, scouring powder, furniture polishes, metal polishes, home dry-cleaning spot removers, toilet bowl cleaners and deodorizers, paints, varnishes, paint removers and strippers, home and garden pesticides, cat litter, flea collars and flea and tick products, interior and exterior cleaners and protectants, car waxes, arts and crafts supplies, typing correction fluids, glues, moth repellent, shoe polishes, cosmetics, hair dye, sunscreens, colorings (food dyes, etc.), synthetic fragrances, dandruff shampoos, hairsprays, mouthwashes, toothpastes and powders, feminine-care body products, bubble baths, and shaving creams. There is also a slight cancer risk associated with the use of electric blankets, and with exposure to electrical goods and wiring that cause low-frequency electromagnetic fields.

Not all brands of the above products contain carcinogenic chemicals; for a definitive list consult *The Safe Shopper's Bible,* by David Steinman and Samuel Epstein (see the Resources section). The authors have made a comprehensive assessment of the chemical contents of almost all Western brands of household goods and have been brave enough to publish it, showing exactly which brands present a potential risk of cancer, hormonal effects, neurotoxicity, and other acute medical problems. A comprehensive list of the offending chemicals to check for can be found in Appendix 2. Be aware that nitrites, which can cause problems in the presence of other chemicals, are often undisclosed or go under the heading of "preservatives."

In general, for nontoxic cleaning, both for people and the environment, Steinman and Epstein recommend the use of the products in the table that follows:

Nontoxic Cleaners

Baking soda (sodium carbonate)	as an excellent cleaner and deodorizer
Beeswax	for polishing
Borax	as a disinfectant
Distilled white vinegar	as an excellent cleaner
Essential oils	to add natural fragrances to homemade cleaning products
Hydrogen peroxide	as a bleach
Lemon juice	as an excellent cleaner
Liquid soap	as an alternative to harsher detergents and cleaning agents
Pumice stone	as a stain remover
Sodium perborate	as an alternative to bleaches made with sodium hypochlorite
Sodium percarbonate	as above
Trisodium phosphate (TSP)	as a powerful cleaning agent
Zeolite	as an excellent deodorizer

(Adapted from David Steinman and Samuel S. Epstein, M.D. The Safe Shopper's Bible. New York: Hungry Minds, Inc., 1995.)

Occupational Exposure
Occupational hazards cause 2 percent of cancer deaths.

The number of occupations in which there is an increased risk of cancer is extensive, and there is a long list of likely or known cancer-producing agents in the workplace (see Appendix 3).

Earlier in the twentieth century, it was estimated that one in twenty-five cancers occurring in the Western/developed world had a major occupational component; but now, with strict control measures in the workplace enforced over the past generation, it is estimated that the number of work-related cancers has halved, at least in developed countries. The key issue for individuals is to know exactly what carcinogenic chemicals are used at their place of work and how they should be handled. The recommended protective clothing should be worn at all times. It is particularly important to find out and observe the rules if you are self-employed. The biggest offenders in this area are likely to be artists, builders, and farmers, who can put themselves at serious risk if they fail to protect themselves properly from the chemicals they are using.

Physical Inactivity
Physical inactivity causes 1.5 percent of cancer deaths.

As long ago as 1912, an Englishman named Rollo Russell said in a book on the preventable causes of cancer that "sedentary occupations are highly injurious for cancer." In the 1980s, men with sedentary occupations were found to be more prone to cancer of the colon. This link prompted further research into the role of exercise in the development of cancer in general. Physical inactivity is now linked to colon, breast, testicular, ovarian, and prostate cancers, and to colon adenoma (which can be precancerous). Exercise may reduce the risk of certain cancers by:

 ❖ decreasing total body fat

 ❖ stimulating immune function

 ❖ favorably affecting hormonal balance

 ❖ speeding up large-intestine transit time (the time it takes for food to pass through the gut)

Certainly in the Eastern model of health and disease, all illness is seen as being related to the stagnation of *chi* (also spelled *qi*) or "vital energy" in the human body. It has been clearly stated that critical damage to genetic material occurs in toxic cellular environments when the concentration of disrupting chemicals reaches a certain level. Exercise is the best way to regularly flush toxins out of the body; thus it comes as no surprise that cancer rates are favorably affected by exercise.

Blood is pumped by the heart through the arteries into the tissues of the body. But when tissue fluids make their way back to the heart through the veins and lymph vessels, there is no pump mechanism other than the muscular movements of the body. As muscles contract during exercise such as walking, bending, or stretching, the tissues are literally "milked," causing the tissue fluid containing toxins to reenter the lymph vessels and veins. From there, toxins are taken to the liver and kidneys to be broken down and eliminated from the body.

This muscular pumping action also helps to bring toxins to the surface of the body, where they are excreted through the skin. You may have noticed the way your sweat smells of curry the day after eating Indian food, or that the sweat of meat eaters is far more pungent than that of vegetarians. These examples show the importance of skin as a route of excretion. Concern has been expressed about the possible role of underarm deodorants in the development of cancer, because many contain strong antiperspirants that block excretion through the skin under the arm. This could, theoretically, result in an accumulation of toxic material in (particularly breast) tissue after prolonged use. However, currently, conventional wisdom holds that this does not constitute a serious health risk.

The lungs also get rid of toxins, by exhaling them. For example, after garlic is eaten, the aroma of garlic on the breath is very noticeable. Many people think the smell comes from the mouth or stomach, but it actually comes directly from the lungs, in the breath. Excretion of toxins via the lungs increases with exercise, as the breathing rate and depth increase.

When people fail to exercise, these vital processes of elimination become severely compromised. I believe that physical inactivity as a cause of cancer may still be underestimated. Certainly, it is likely to play a significant role as people grow older. Until recently, it was not unusual for people over the age of thirty with Western lifestyles to get no exercise at all apart from an occasional walk. But fortunately, this trend has changed over the past thirty years. The recognition of the importance of exercise in preventing heart disease gave sports and exercise a big boost, resulting in the jogging craze of the 1970s and 1980s. Since then, general emphasis on the "body beautiful" has led to a wholesale return of people of all age groups to the gym and to fitness or dance classes in pursuit of both the perfect physique and the greatly improved well-being and vitality that accompany serious exercise.

Another interesting observation is that cancer occurs more often in the left breast than in the right. As the majority of women are right-handed, it stands to reason that the right arm and breast are being moved and exercised more than the left. Indeed, many women carry a great deal of tension in their left shoulder and arm, holding the left arm closer to the body than the right one, effectively limiting the flow of blood and lymph under the left arm. For this reason it is a good idea to check regularly for tension in the left arm and shoulder (or in the right if you are left-handed) and also to stretch your arms above your head several times a day.

Scientific evidence even suggests that wearing a bra increases the risk of breast cancer. One of the early signs of breast cancer that can be seen on a CAT scan or ultrasound is the presence of calcium deposits within the breast tissue. This occurs where the tissue becomes "stagnant" (in Chinese terms), allowing the buildup of these chalky deposits. When a woman wears a bra, especially an under-wire bra, less movement of the breast occurs; this may slow down the toxin-clearing process from the breast. However, breast cancer incidence increases with both a larger breast size and the wearing of bras, and this may have muddled the research findings. More research is therefore needed before definitive advice can be given about the safety of bras.

Medical Procedures
Medical procedures cause 0.5 percent of cancer deaths.

It is disturbing to learn that medical procedures can themselves be a cause of cancer deaths. Paradoxically, all the treatments for cancer are themselves carcinogenic. Quite frequently, if a person with cancer is fortunate enough to survive the disease, a second, quite different cancer can develop in another part of the body because of the carcinogenic effects of chemotherapy and radiation therapy. In this situation the new cancer is not a secondary of the old one, but a different cancer altogether that has been triggered by the treatments. For example, tamoxifen, the estrogen-blocking drug commonly used to help improve the prognosis of breast cancer, carries a 5–10 percent risk of causing endometrial (uterine-lining) cancer.

Birth control pills and hormone replacement therapy increase the risk of cancer, and repeated X rays, CAT scans, and magnetic-resonance imaging (MRI), and possibly repeated ultrasound scans, are also linked to the development of the disease. All of these tests involve exposing the body to electromagnetic radiation, which at high levels can cause cancer—particularly in susceptible individuals. As mentioned previously, abdominal X rays of pregnant women are estimated to cause 5 percent of childhood leukemia.

Obviously, great care must be taken to keep medical radiation exposure within safe limits. But it is difficult to be sure what the safe limit is for a given patient, especially when confounding factors such as occupational exposure, poor diet, smoking, or a genetic predisposition may exist.

Cancerous tumors are also more likely to develop in people on immunosuppressive drugs, which are required after organ transplantation. Typically, these patients are more likely to develop lymphoma. Other, rarer cancers also exist that can be triggered by medical procedures, drugs, and tests.

The fact that modern medicine can cause cancer is a very good incentive to try to *prevent* disease; with this in mind, it is advisable to avoid medical testing and drugs unless they are absolutely necessary and as safe as possible. Take the time to quiz the members of your health-care team closely about the possible side effects of all the drugs, tests, and treatments you are offered; this includes your primary physician as well as any specialists, such as radiologists, who treat you. Many hospitals or clinics now offer an "ask-a-nurse" phone line for just this sort of question.

Cancer and the Mind

Let us return to the topic of the mind/body connection in cancer, introduced earlier in the chapter. The notion that state of mind is somehow linked to the chance of getting cancer has been around for centuries. In the second century a.d., the Greek physician Galen said, "Melancholic women are more prone to cancer than sanguine women." In 1800, an eminent doctor named Walshe pointed to "the influence of mental misery, sudden reverse of fortune and habitual gloomings of temper on the disposition of carcinomatous matter." And in 1870, Paget noted that "deep mental distress is among the conditions favorable to the occurrence of cancer." During the mid-1900s, the concept of a "cancer personality" emerged.

People thought to be especially prone to cancer were those who were unable to express hostile feelings, had a rigid personality and a tendency toward social conformity (doing what was expected of them by society), lacked self-awareness, had a tendency toward introspection, self-blame, and feelings of hopelessness and despair, and were likely to have few outlets for their emotions.

Psychologist Lawrence LeShan refined this concept in the 1960s and 1970s. He found that the lives of people who get cancer are marked by feelings of isolation, neglect, and despair during childhood, followed by relationship problems and the development of a consuming interest (either in a strong and meaningful relationship or in a satisfying vocation) that becomes the center of their life as an adult. Loss of this relationship or role results in despair, reactivating the painful feelings of childhood.

LeShan found that these people were also more likely to bottle up despair and to be "kind, sweet and benign" while hiding feelings of anger, hurt, and hostility.

Over time, the same themes have kept recurring, with the strong suggestion that stress, bottled-up emotions, traumatic life events, isolation, and depression are linked to cancer, or certainly to a worse prognosis in cancer.

However, during the late 1980s and the 1990s, conventional scientific research into the role of stress and life events on cancer has been conflicting. While some studies show positive associations, others do not. But we should resist discounting a theory too quickly that has been around for so long. It seems likely that further research will show that it is not stress as such that affects physical health, but rather how well or how poorly different individuals cope with it.

When considering psychological influences on cancer, several factors need to be taken into account. First, cancer rates are higher among those who are isolated, depressed, or socially disadvantaged—and such sufferers also die sooner. Of course, there are many aspects of being socially disadvantaged, such as poor nutrition, that could lead to an increased risk of cancer. But it is also very common that socially disadvantaged individuals are disempowered and lack creative expression, and therefore feel frustrated and depressed as a result.

Second, in the 1980s there was strong evidence from the eminent psychosocial oncologist Dr. Stephen Greer that people with cancer who have a strong "fighting spirit" survive much longer with the same cancer than those who become "helpless and hopeless." Other studies show that patients who receive help in a support group to express their negative feelings also survive longer. These groups help patients to express their anger, grief, fear, and despair, and this act of emotional expression carries a very significant survival benefit.

Third, patients who practice the mind/body technique of visualization (imagining positive outcomes to treatment) while undergoing chemotherapy for cancer also enjoy better survival rates. In this technique, once patients are relaxed and during the actual treatment, they are instructed to visualize a series of positive images of the benefits they should receive from chemotherapy. Studies also show that people with very high social conformity benefit particularly profoundly in terms of long-term survival, having a 13 percent improvement in survival rate fifteen years after the intervention.

Fourth, on an anecdotal level, anyone involved in the care of people with cancer will tell you that when patients lose their will to live, death can follow very quickly, no matter what medicine, orthodox or complementary, is being given. There is even research from the United States showing that difficult patients survive longer! Another interesting phenomenon is that while more women get breast cancer in the United States than in the UK, fewer die of it. Medics believe this has to do with better screening or medicine in the States, but my own hunch is that it may well be due to the far more assertive, upbeat reaction of most Americans and their doctors to diagnosis and illness management, and to lower levels of depression and far higher levels of fighting spirit. By contrast, the response to cancer diagnosis in the UK is often very passive and gloomy, with many doctors tending to crush patients' efforts to fight the disease rather than encouraging attempts at self-help.

All this evidence suggests strongly that one's state of mind definitely affects the progress of cancer growth in the body, although it still seems unlikely that particular states of mind will ever be shown to be an actual cause of cancer. What does seem likely is that negative states of mind have a direct effect on the immune system and tissue functioning, weakening the body's defenses against cancer. The new field of psychoneuroimmunology (PNI) looks at the connection between our minds, hormonal systems, and the functioning of the immune system and tissues of the body. It has shown, without any shadow of doubt, that stress definitely alters the activity not only of the immune system but also of all other tissues. What has been found is that receptors exist on all the cells of the body for brain messenger chemicals called *neuropeptides*, which, when activated, can either excite or depress cell functioning.

In those who are stressed and depressed, immune and other tissue functioning can be markedly depressed too, influencing both the number of circulating immune cells and their individual activity. This can put people at risk of infections and other illnesses, and it is very likely that prolonged stress or severe shock and upset can allow abnormal cancer cells (which would normally be spotted and destroyed) to escape surveillance and survive. However, the degree of cellular and immune-system depression varies greatly among individuals who experience similar levels of stress. It now appears clear from other psychological and PNI studies that the key determinant is not how much stress or upset we have but how we respond to it.

The immune system is able to learn responses and to become programmed to key triggers. Thus it is likely that those who are sensitized early in life to loss, grief, powerlessness, and anxiety, and who suppress their emotional response to these problems, have a particularly pronounced psychological and immunological reaction to subsequent problems. Some people will therefore be more at risk due to their psychological makeup and history. This may well be the reason why population studies do not show clear-cut results in relation to stress and adverse life events and cancer incidence. However, it is more likely that the general increase in stress in society from high-pressure living is weakening our immune systems and may be a significant factor in the increasing incidence of cancer. This picture of individualized stress-risk factors parallels the situation with chemicals and cancer—there are chemicals that affect us all but that are particularly risky to those with a specific vulnerability to them.

In time, no doubt the true extent of the risks created by psychological factors will be known and the potential role of the mind in helping us to survive and prevent cancer will be understood. It will not be long before we are able to screen and monitor individuals for the effects of stress on their body tissue and immune function. Using this information, we will be able to offer protective psychological strategies to those who are especially vulnerable. In the meantime, because of this new scientific work and the experience of the Bristol Cancer Help Centre and other cancer support centers, we currently have enough understanding of the huge importance of psychological health and mind/body techniques in cancer to reasonably include the mind/body element in advice on cancer prevention.

It is clear from these statistics how much the risk of cancer increases over the age of sixty-five. With life expectancy increasing all the time, we must all take steps now to prevent cancer when we are older, so that our potentially golden years do not become a misery.

RISK FACTORS FOR SPECIFIC CANCERS

There is considerable variation in the risk factors for different cancers. A list of the risk factors for the most common cancers can be found in Appendix 4.

Who Is at Risk?

With the emphasis that has been put over the past decade on the importance of genetic factors in the development of cancer, the public could not be blamed for thinking that the disease is largely an inherited one. However, as I have shown, a family history of cancer accounts for only between 1 and 5 percent of all cancers. Even in this small group of genetic cancers, we need to ask ourselves if or how much lifestyle and environmental pollution play a part in activating cancer genes. Cancer genes have always existed, and it is likely that it is our poor diet and toxic lifestyles that are now causing the oncogenes to express themselves increasingly frequently. Don't forget: Even cancer-prone genes still need to undergo at least one or two mutations before they become activated oncogenes or "cancer genes." It is therefore important that we avoid falling into a sense of impotence, thinking that cancer is an inherited disease about which we can do very little.

As of the year 2001, eleven cancer-prone genes had been discovered that are involved in normal cell growth and division and that can, if mutated, lead to the development of chronic myeloid leukemia; lymphoid neoplasms; chronic lymphatic leukemia; Burkitt's lymphoma; cancer of the breast, ovaries, bladder, stomach, lung, cervix, colon, pancreas, genitourinary tract, and thyroid; squamous head and neck tumors; melanomas (skin cancer); and endocrine (or glandular) cancers.

There are an additional seventeen tumor-suppressor genes that, if mutated, can become involved in the development of cancers of the colon, duodenum (small intestine), lymph, breast, ovaries, prostate, pancreas, uterus, urinary tract, kidney, brain and thyroid; pheochromocytoma (cancer of the adrenal gland), sarcomas (cancers of the bones or connective tissues), melanomas, leukemias, retinoblastoma (tumor of the retina, in the back of the eye), osteosarcoma, and hemangioblastoma (cancer of the bloodvessel walls). Despite this huge list of cancers in which oncogenes can be implicated, it is important to remember that most cancers

Which Are the Most Common Cancers?

In men [UK]:

Type of Cancer	% by age 65	Over lifetime	Lifetime risk
Lung	1.7	8.0	1 in 13
Prostate	0.9	7.3	1 in 14
Colorectal	1.4	5.7	1 in 18
Bladder	0.7	3.3	1 in 30
Stomach	0.5	2.3	1 in 44
Esophageal	0.4	1.3	1 in 75
Kidney	0.4	1.1	1 in 89
Leukemia	0.4	1.1	1 in 94
Pancreatic	0.3	1.0	1 in 96

In women [UK]:

Type of Cancer	% by age 65	Over lifetime	Lifetime risk
Breast	5.6	10.9	1 in 9
Colorectal	1.1	4.9	1 in 20
Lung	0.4	4.3	1 in 23
Ovarian	0.9	2.1	1 in 48
Uterine	0.6	1.4	1 in 73
Bladder	0.2	1.3	1 in 79
Stomach	0.2	1.2	1 in 86
Pancreatic	0.2	1.1	1 in 95
Cervical	0.6	0.9	1 in 116

(Statistics from The Cancer Registry *[UK], 1997.)*

arise from the longer five- or six-step process that occurs in previously normal tissue (described above in the section titled "What Is Cancer?").

From this chapter's overview of the causes of cancer, it is clear that a combination of occupation and lifestyle can have a big influence on one's likelihood of getting the disease. Overall, the factor that increases the incidence of cancer the most is age. The longer we live, the more our chance of developing cancer increases dramatically. This is due to a combination of many of the factors already mentioned—the accumulation of toxins in the body over time, leading to an increase in genetic mutation; decreasing physical activity; obesity; hormone replacement therapy; medical procedures; smoking; alcohol; and, in general, a decrease in the reliability of cellular function and regulatory mechanisms, especially when nutrition is poor, with an over-processed, over-rich Western diet.

Because modern medicine and health improvements enable people to live longer, we now have a society with a large number of elderly people. As the population ages, there is an associated rise in cancer incidence and, therefore, mortality. However, there are also worrisome increases in cancer incidence among younger people, especially smoking-related cancers in women and childhood leukemias.

The other major factors that affect cancer incidence are nationality, culture, and social and societal trends. In fact, it has been the study of this disease in different populations that has shed so much light on the causes of cancer and the possibility of preventing it. It is not easy to persuade people to change or to get societies to adopt wholesale the values and customs of others. However, gaining insight from the differing patterns of cancer incidence around the world can give us a vital starting place to understand the most important factors.

A good example of national variations can be seen in Japanese people living in Japan, who have high stomach cancer rates but very low rates of breast cancer compared with people in the West. In the UK and the United States, a woman has around a one-in-nine lifetime chance of developing breast cancer, whereas in Japan it is closer to one in forty-five. This has been attributed to the far lower incidence of obesity in Japanese women; the lower circulating levels of postmenopausal estrogen; the extremely low intake of dairy foods and relatively low intake of meat, along with a high intake of soy products (which contain phytoestrogens); and the drinking of green tea. Phytoestrogens are very weak estrogenic compounds that sit on and block cells' estrogen hormone receptors, acting a bit like tamoxifen, the estrogen-blocking drug. This is thought to protect Japanese women from the effects of circulating estrogen, thus conveying significant protection against breast cancer. On the other hand, the Japanese diet includes large amounts of protein (particularly in the form of raw fish) as well as vegetable pickles and salted foods. These predispose the Japanese to a high level of stomach cancer.

Sadly, once Japanese women forsake their traditional culture for a Western lifestyle, their protection against breast cancer is lost. Japanese people who move to the United States, for example, develop the lower stomach cancer and higher breast cancer rates of American Caucasians within only five years of arriving.

In some developing countries, cancer is much more likely to be caused by infectious agents, and it is already known that liver cancer is associated with the intake of aflatoxin. It is also clear that in Africa, where rural communities eat mainly high-fiber vegetarian diets, there are very low levels of both hormonal and gastric cancers. On the other hand, sexually transmitted cancers, such as cervical cancer, are far more common.

The gravest concern for the developing world is that posed by the wholesale adoption of Western lifestyles. People within traditional cultures need to be informed as a matter of urgency about the severe health risks associated with a Western lifestyle and diet and given strong reinforcement of the healthy aspects of their traditional lifestyles. There is a great risk that the media image of Western success will overtake and smother traditional values, wiping out many unique cultures and placing many people's health at great risk.

For the Western world, the challenge is to prevent a significant rise in viral cancers of the cervix, liver, and blood caused by a combination of poor nutrition, poverty, drug addiction (through the use of nonsterile needles), and unsafe sex.

CONVENTIONAL CANCER TREATMENT

Despite the billions of pounds and dollars that have been poured into cancer research over the past fifty years and the enormous increase in our understanding of the way cancer develops, medical treatment still remains woefully ineffective in offering hope of a cure to the majority of people with the disease. Realistically, the possibility of a cure can be offered only to those with three of the relatively rarer cancers—testicular cancer, some of the lymphomas, and some leukemias.

Cancer medicine does not greatly alter the long-term prognosis in any of the common cancers (of the lung, breast, bowel, and prostate), where the major role of conventional treatment is to delay spread of the disease and to increase what is known as the "disease-free interval." This means symptoms and signs of the illness are temporarily removed so the patient can enjoy a relatively normal life for longer, until the return of the disease eventually makes death inevitable. Newer medical approaches are beginning to offer some promising increases in life expectancy, but compared to the amount of work that has gone into trying to achieve these ends, the results are disappointing. The conventional treatments for cancer typically include:

❖ surgery, to remove the tumor (where it is a solid tumor rather than a blood cancer)

❖ radiotherapy, where radiation is used after surgery to destroy stray cells around the operation site that may have been missed during surgery, or to treat inoperable cancers or cancer secondaries that may be causing severe local problems such as nerve or arterial compression

❖ chemotherapy, which involves giving drugs that destroy rapidly dividing cells (rapid division is the main feature distinguishing cancer cells from other cells, although other rapidly dividing tissue such as skin, nails, hair, the gut lining, and immune and other blood cells may also be damaged in the process)

❖ adjuvant hormone-blocking therapy, given in cancers of the breast and prostate to block female and male hormones that stimulate a tumor's growth

It is the relative lack of efficacy of cancer medicine and the very rigorous nature of these treatments (which in themselves can produce secondary cancers) that make the issue of prevention so vital. For this reason, and because cancer is such a serious and unpleasant disease, it is imperative that the prevention and eradication of cancer move to the top of our personal, professional, and societal agendas.

THE STATE OF CANCER RESEARCH

The majority of the cancer research budget in the United States, the UK, and mainland Europe is currently dedicated to investigating how cancer develops and to the treatment of cancer. A very small proportion of the budget is spent on researching prevention or, more importantly, on the implementation of cancer prevention strategies. We already have enough key information to eradicate a large proportion of preventable cancer. For one, the American National Breast Cancer Coalition has discovered that women with breast cancer feel that the highest priority for cancer research should be prevention, not treatment.

At present, by far the biggest proportion of cancer research budgets worldwide goes into research on the role of genetics in cancer formation. The hope is that by understanding properly how cancer develops, doctors will be able to formulate better treatment strategies. Currently, on the treatment side, a lot of work is focused on developing mechanisms to target chemotherapy drugs that will work only on the cancer itself and not affect other tissues. Work is also underway to see if genetically modified viruses can be used to correct genetic abnormalities in cancer cells, as well as other techniques to repair defective DNA. Many other trials are comparing the efficacy of different mixtures and types of chemotherapy drugs.

The other big push currently among UK cancer-research charities is for studies in the use of the hormone-blocking drug tamoxifen to prevent breast cancer in healthy women. As mentioned earlier, this avenue of research also has its opponents.

Almost weekly we see press reports of important cancer breakthroughs, but in reality these usually amount to tiny clues in a massive jigsaw puzzle. They are often laboratory findings in animal studies that may or may not be found to relate to human cancer development or treatment.

Encouragingly, in the UK, a large-scale trial—the European Prospective Investigation into Cancer and Nutrition—is looking in depth at the relationship between diet and cancer. In the UK alone, twenty-five thousand men and women have been recruited for this study, and their dietary patterns and cancer incidence will be compared with that of a further four hundred thousand people in mainland Europe in order to assess the incidence of cancer in relation to different eating patterns. Another study is looking at whether a daily intake of the mineral selenium can reduce cancer incidence. This link is being investigated because more cancer cases occur in areas where the soil is lower in selenium; early findings are promising.

In the United States, the potential role of alternative and complementary therapies is also being taken seriously at last. The government-run National Institutes of Health has set up an Office of Alternative Medicines, which in turn is currently setting up research centers for all areas of medicine. The center for the study of alternative and complementary medicine in cancer is located at the University of Texas M. D. Anderson Cancer Center in Houston. There, they are studying the effectiveness of different herbs, vitamins, mineral supplements, and foods when used with orthodox treatment, as well as studying them in their own right for cancer treatment and palliative care.

The reality of the situation, as stated in 1998 by Professor Karol Sikora, formerly of the World Health Organization's Department of Cancer Strategy, is that it is unlikely that the *treatment* of cancer will ever be the solution to the problem. We must therefore wake up and focus all our efforts on cancer prevention and heed the message given to us by the rising incidence of cancer about our societal and environmental problems. We must look forward with hope to the great personal and social rewards of tackling cancer at its source. We must refuse to passively accept cancer as a part of life while we watch the effects of this dreadful Western disease spread inexorably among our friends and family, and into developing countries that lack resources to deal with the problem.

It is also important to recognize that while the public relations messages of the cancer organizations, telling us of the great breakthroughs being made daily, are vital to their own survival and ongoing work (important and laudable as those may be), they might keep us focused on the wrong priorities—those of cause and treatment rather than prevention. We must not hope just to *treat* cancer; we must hope to *eradicate* it, and the way to do that is through cancer prevention.

CANCER POLITICS

If you were a shaper of public policy today, faced with the reality that cancer is a problem created by cigarettes, Western diet, alcohol, the chemical industry, intensive farming, and environmental pollution, not to mention the medical profession, you might feel ever so slightly daunted by the prospect of trying to eradicate it. To take on the combined might of the tobacco, alcohol, pharmaceutical, petrochemical, and agricultural industries, plus the medical profession, would be immediate political suicide for any politician.

During the heat of the initial bovine spongiform encephalopathy (BSE, or mad-cow disease) crisis in the mid-1990s, the British Committee on the Medical Aspects of Food was also reviewing evidence about the relationship between cancer and diet. The findings of Doctors T. J. Key and M. Thorogood—that vegetarians were

40 to 50 percent less likely to die of cancer than meat eaters—had been published in 1994, but it took this committee until 1998 to make the public recommendation that meat eating was definitely associated with increased cancer risk. Not surprisingly, the release of the committee's findings was not made public until the heat had gone out of the first wave of the BSE crisis.

In 1996, when asked face to face why the British government was not taking a more direct approach to the link between cancer and diet, the then Secretary of State for Health replied quite unashamedly, "How could we—the farmers would kill us!"

It is difficult for any government with a short term of office and its eye on the next election to make the kinds of decisions that will truly protect the health of the nation. Successive governments focus on achieving health targets through the improvement of medicine rather than tackling the core root of the problem of degenerative illness. It is likely that while medicine is firmly in the grip of the pharmaceutical companies and governments are firmly in the hands of industry and market forces, we will never see policies being made that address the problem of cancer head-on. Instead, present-day governments focus on small-scale movements seeking to increase health awareness within the community that puts the responsibility for leading healthy lives back into our own hands.

This means that it is up to all of us as individuals to take charge ourselves—in our family group, in our places of work, in our institutions and local communities—and to put in place, step by step, the behavioral changes, policies, and practices that will systematically eradicate cancer from our lives and from our society. As more and more healthy-living initiatives develop, giving support particularly to the most disadvantaged in society, the great hope is that the public will be empowered and enabled to make healthy choices, and that the incidence of cancer will drop steadily over the years to come.

2

❖

Cleaning Up Your Act

This chapter contains specific advice on how to eliminate potential causes of cancer from your life. Considerable emphasis is given to getting the necessary support and help to change the habits of a lifetime, especially when these habits represent emotional crutches "to get you through the day," such as unhealthy use of food, alcohol, or cigarettes.

The main issues to address in relation to food and cancer are:

❖ obesity

❖ foods and food additives

❖ cooking methods

OBESITY

Obesity has already been linked to an increased risk of cancer of the breast, endometrium (uterine lining), gallbladder, and large intestine, and is likely to be linked to cancer of the prostate, ovaries, kidney, and pancreas.

Obesity is measured by calculating body mass index, or BMI (see page 24 for information on how to calculate BMI). The World Health Organization (WHO) defines obesity as a BMI greater than thirty, overweight as a BMI of twenty-five or above, and desirable weight as a BMI of between twenty and twenty-five.

World Health Organization Weight Categories

BMI:	20–24.9	25–29.9	30–40	greater than 40
Description:	desirable weight	overweight	obese	severely obese

Obesity levels in developed countries are rising at alarming rates. The United States has the worst obesity record. At least thirty-nine million Americans are obese: more than one-fourth of all adults and about one in five children. (A full 55 percent of adult Americans—ninety-seven million—are categorized as overweight or obese.) The number of overweight and obese Americans has risen steadily since 1960, and this trend continues.

In the UK, the obesity problem has increased dramatically over the last two decades. In 1980, 8 percent of women and 6 percent of men were obese; today, those rates have risen to 21.2 percent and 17.3 percent respectively. This means that in only twenty years the prevalence of obesity in the UK has almost tripled.

Obesity is a risk factor not only for cancer. People who are overweight are at higher risk for all the degenerative diseases—especially those of the cardiovascular system and joints. Hopefully, by understanding that obesity is a serious risk factor for cancer as well as heart disease, you will feel compelled, if necessary, to do something about your own weight, your diet, and, if possible, about the diet of those in your immediate sphere of influence.

In developing countries, obesity is associated with affluence, and obesity may even be considered desirable. However, the opposite is true in developed countries. Obesity rates are much higher in the lower socioeconomic classes than in professional groups. In the UK, for example, serious obesity levels increase from 10.7 percent among the well-off to 25.3 percent among those living in poverty.

To tackle the issue globally, the International Obesity Task Force (IOTF) was formed under the auspices of the WHO (see the Resources section). The IOTF's aims are:

❖ to raise awareness at all levels that obesity is a serious medical condition and a major global health problem

❖ to develop policy recommendations for a coherent and effective global approach to managing and preventing obesity

❖ to identify and implement strategies in collaboration with experts, professional organizations, patient groups, and national health agencies

Tackling the Personal Problem of Excess Weight

Finding out if you are overweight or obese is the first step to tackling the problem. You may wish to calculate your BMI (see page 24) and determine which of the WHO categories you fall into (see the table on the previous page). This will give you a clear indication of how urgent the problem is for you personally.

If your BMI is in the obese or severely obese category, you may be able to receive help and support in losing weight from your family doctor or a weight-loss clinic. Other options exist as well. Getting the right sort of help is discussed starting on page 75, in the section titled "How We Eat."

Even if you are overweight rather than obese, I urge you strongly to act now to take your weight and diet in hand. While it is extremely important not to let your self-esteem suffer as a result of being overweight, it is vital for your health, well-being, and quality of life that this issue be tackled head-on. In addition to considering your own weight, it is important to extend your concern about healthy eating and the avoidance of obesity to places of work, schools, hospitals, prisons, and nursing homes. If you are involved in the management of any of these organizations or use any of these facilities, get involved in making sure that the organization makes the adoption of a healthy eating policy a priority. A good place to start is by replacing easy access to sweets, chips, or sugary drinks with access to fruit, fruit juices, whole-food snacks, and bottled water.

The Causes of Obesity

In a few rare situations, the causes of obesity are medical. But for the vast majority of us, obesity is caused by or results from:

❖ the foods we eat

❖ how much we eat

❖ how we eat

The Foods We Eat

Fat, Sugar, and Alcohol. Dietary fat, refined sugars, and alcohol are the biggest contributors to the onset of obesity. Many people in developed countries in effect double their calorie intake each day by eating sweets or fatty snacks such as chips, or by drinking sugary drinks or alcohol. None of these things contribute to our body's well-being or our overall good health. Instead, they make us fat and lethargic and put our health at risk. Another problem is that they contain empty calories that satisfy our hunger and thus reduce our appetite for healthy foods that contain the essential vitamins, minerals, and plant phytochemicals required for protection against cancer. A further problem is that a sudden rise in sugar, fat, or alcohol levels in the bloodstream puts the body under physiological stress, and all tissue function (particularly that of the brain) is potentially lethally threatened. The body's rebalancing mechanisms then have to work very hard to restore equilibrium, a process that uses up a lot of precious vitamins and minerals.

So by snacking on junk food, people can end up both obese and depleted in vital nutrients. Growing children, the sick, and the elderly are at greatest risk because they are often more tempted by sweet foods and soft drinks that have virtually no nutritional value, only empty calories. These nutrition-poor foods particularly affect our overall growth, brain development, the aging process, and our resistance to disease.

Fried Foods. The next biggest contributor to obesity is fried food, whether eaten at home or in fast-food outlets. It is virtually impossible to buy healthy food in fast-food restaurants, where the main emphasis is on burgers, french fries, and snacks covered in batter and breadcrumbs, such as chicken nuggets. To make things worse, most children's meals from fast-food outlets include no vegetables other than fries. (As mentioned earlier, it has been estimated that 47 percent of inner-city children in the UK eat no vegetables other than fries.)

Often, adults who cook vegetables and make salads for themselves feed their children a regular diet of burgers, chicken fingers, and pizza. These might be washed down with a soft drink and followed by ice cream. We then wonder why so many children become sickly, irritable, and obese, and why they underachieve at school!

Animal Fats and Meat. The emphasis on meat and animal fats in the Western diet also plays a major role in obesity. Heavy consumption of cheese, meat, butter, cream, and yogurt has disastrous consequences on our health and weight. In Asian cultures, where there is a far higher intake of rice, grains, and vegetables, with protein and animal fat used only in smaller quantities, obesity is practically nonexistent.

How Much We Eat

Figuring out how much we eat—both at meal times and in snacks—is an important first step in tackling obesity. Keeping a food diary for a week is one way to monitor eating patterns. When you see the amount you eat written down in black and white, it can be quite shocking. Because access to snacks at home, at work, and on the street is so easy for most people these days—not to mention the almost twenty-four-hour availability of sweets and soft drinks in supermarkets, movie theatres, and convenience stores—it is easy to be munching all the time. Guidelines for good health indicate that children should have around 1,750 calories a day, women around 2,000, and men around 2,500 if they have a fairly sedentary lifestyle, often the norm in this day and age. The total calories required will vary according to the height and occupation of the person. In an affluent Western diet it is easy to consume in excess of the entire daily calorie allowance in one meal. For example, by starting with cocktails and peanuts, moving on to an hors d'oeuvre such as pâté with bread and butter, tucking into a main meal such as steak and fries, enjoying cheesecake for dessert, topping it off with coffee and chocolates, and washing everything down with a couple glasses of wine or pints of beer, you would consume 3,750 calories! A child who consumes two bags of chips, three canned soft drinks, and a chocolate bar will have consumed 1,000 calories without any proper food at all.

It also seems true that the more we eat the more we *want* to eat. We get used to eating large meals on a regular basis, and as portions get larger, the amount we need to eat to feel satisfied gets larger, and the vicious circle continues. People's awareness that they tend to eat excessively during the evening or when they go out may lead to another problem—the diet/binge phenomenon. People may starve themselves all day so they can go out and eat a huge meal in the evening. Much evidence exists to suggest that this type of famine-and-feast routine is counterproductive in terms of putting on weight. In response to the famine phase our bodies go into a very low and efficient basal metabolic rate, maintaining our weight by burning calories very slowly. Then, as the calories come rushing in during the feast, the body goes straight into a fat-storage mode in case more famine is on the way! It is therefore definitely not a good idea to adopt this type of strategy for weight control. Evidence also shows that if we eat the majority of our calories at the end of the day, when there is no chance to exercise and burn them off, more fat is deposited throughout the night than would be if the equivalent amount of food were eaten at breakfast or lunchtime.

When we snack or "graze" continuously, we hardly ever feel hungry. On the other hand, when we eat very large meals, we become used to overriding feelings of fullness and satisfaction and go on eating beyond what we actually need. To become healthy it is important to start over: Tune into yourself and learn what your body really needs, rather than eating too much out of habit.

To avoid obesity:

❖ Reduce the amount of calories in each meal, keeping within the daily calorie allowance.

❖ Avoid snacks between meals other than fresh fruit, vegetables, and whole-food snacks such as whole-grain crackers and low-fat granola bars.

❖ Eat regular meals, spreading calorie intake evenly throughout the day.

❖ Avoid eating the bulk of your calories at the end of the day.

How We Eat

For many people in the West, consumption of food has come to have very little to do with hunger. Much of what we eat is either for sensory gratification (to provide emotional comfort or sedation, or to cover nervousness) or in social contexts. Rich, fatty foods temporarily dampen anxiety and emotional stress because blood flow to the digestive system is prioritized away from the brain and muscles. This is why we feel sleepy after a big meal and are advised not to swim soon after eating. There is nothing wrong with food being a source of sensory delight, but it is vital that we learn how to choose and cook foods low in calories and that are good for us. This kind of food can be made equally delightful once we acquire the necessary knowledge and develop the right skills. Chapter 4 explains in great detail how to go about converting an unhealthy eating style to a healthy one—without losing any of the appeal and satisfaction.

The emotional and social factors that determine what we eat are far more difficult to confront. Many people are aware that they "comfort eat" when they are lonely, depressed, or anxious. Others comfort eat without realizing what they are doing. Family or institutional regimens with set meal times and set menus of many courses can cause people to adopt a way of eating that does not necessarily suit their constitution or appetite. In a family situation, pushy relatives may repeatedly urge their partner or dependents to eat more than they would otherwise, deriving satisfaction (and an element of control) from this caregiving role. In the process, their loved ones become overweight, sedated, and addicted to the wrong foods.

Another factor of the general Western eating style is that eating and drinking have become major recreational activities. As recently as a generation ago, a meal out was a special occasion. But today, eating out for many people is a weekly if not daily event. This has created a new kind of emotional dependence on food— the feeling that you haven't had a good time unless socializing has included the consumption of food.

Changing our emotional and social eating patterns takes enormous focus and determination and a great deal of support. This is why most attempts to change people's health patterns simply through health promotion fail. Many people have the necessary information about what is good or bad for them but lack sufficient motivation or support to make the required changes.

The Emotional Element. To find out if there is a major emotional element to your way of eating, consider whether you:

- eat more when you are anxious, depressed, or lonely;

- feel really bad if you cannot get access to food;

- reward yourself with food when you have done something difficult;

- get anxious if food is late or if there is a possibility that someone else will eat the food allocated to you;

- binge on certain foods at times or have rituals and routines around shopping and food.

In simple terms, the use of food for comfort eating is linked to a need for emotional contact, love, support, touch, communication, and security. The way to change an unhealthy dependency on food is to find ways of meeting these underlying needs directly, rather than indirectly by eating.

Sometimes the link between emotions and foods goes beyond mere comfort eating and moves into the realm of an eating disorder. This can result in someone becoming either overweight or, more commonly, underweight. If this is the case with you and you feel your eating habits are out of control, ruling your life, or endangering you in some way, it may be time to seek psychological or psychiatric help, as well as help to bring your weight under control. Once you can recognize that you use food in an unhealthy and detrimental manner and reach out for the help and support you need, the problem can eventually be sorted out.

It may be possible to do this by yourself if you have good friends, a concerned family, or a helpful partner who are willing and able to give you the support and love you need. However, especially if you are isolated and even if you are not, you may need the help of a professional counselor or support group to learn to deal with your emotional needs in a different, healthier way. There are a great number of support groups available that are dedicated to helping people lose weight; the most well known is Weight Watchers (see the Resources section). Some group programs focus mainly on dietary regimens with goals and rewards for losing weight, while others are more psychologically oriented, attempting to help participants learn to fill the gap left by letting go of excessive food consumption. One of these is Overeaters Anonymous, whose methods are based on the twelve steps of Alcoholics Anonymous. As with AA, attendance at OA is free, but a basket is passed at each meeting to collect voluntary donations for covering basic expenses (see the Resources section). Other groups focus on the use of a product to help with appetite suppression so you don't need to eat so much. However, if the underlying emotional needs remain unaddressed, these techniques will only be a temporary solution. Getting help from a counselor and joining the right kind of support group is usually the surest way to make real, long-term changes.

The other way to help yourself emotionally is to approach the problem from the opposite direction by working on your emotional state through the use of self-help techniques such as relaxation, meditation, yoga, and tai chi. These techniques help to calm the mind and emotions and enable you to develop inner peace and strength. Once your mind is calmer, stronger, and more peaceful, you will enjoy far more control and choice over how you behave. Developing some sort of exercise routine also will help psychologically and physically, lifting your emotional state while burning up unwanted calories. Again, you may have the discipline and support to exercise on your own, but if sticking with a fitness plan is a challenge, find a partner or buddy to do it with you. For couples, a healthy active sex life is also helpful, both physically and mentally.

The Social Element. Changing the social aspect of our eating habits also requires a strong commitment. It may well involve confronting a partner or parent who continually urges you to eat more. It may mean taking a good look at yourself and the way you feed others. If someone else cooks for you and won't change their way of cooking, then you need to exert great self-discipline by eating only appropriate amounts of suitable foods. This can be hurtful and difficult for both the provider and you, but it may be the only way to show them that you are serious. Hopefully, in the long term, your taking a stand will prompt them to change their behavior, too.

When hosting a party, it is hard to change one's eating patterns without thinking you are depriving your guests or being a poor host or hostess. Thus, party planning requires a great deal of imagination, and perhaps even frank discussion with friends about what you are trying to do. A good start is to plan social events around an activity other than eating. For example, you could get together with friends to enjoy music, poetry, sports, games, a film or play, or even to meditate together. Of course, you can still provide some sort of refreshments, but as they will be the secondary rather than the primary focus, food consumption will be much lower. This may be a tougher task for women than for men, as many women define themselves partly by their role as cooks and hostesses; they will need to find new ways to express their creativity and generosity.

So, to correct both the emotional and social elements of how you eat:

❖ Ascertain if you are eating to fulfill emotional needs, and if so, find ways to meet these needs more appropriately.

❖ Emphasize the activities that constitute your social gatherings, not the refreshments.

FOODS AND FOOD ADDITIVES THAT
INCREASE CANCER RISK

The main foods to eliminate from your diet in order to decrease the
risk of cancer are:

❖ red meat (pork, beef, lamb)

❖ animal fats

❖ foods that are pickled, preserved, smoked, or salted

❖ food additives

Red Meat

The Western diet is very protein-rich, with meals at home and in
restaurants often focused on large pieces of meat or fish with few
vegetables other than for decoration. There has been a dramatic
rise in meat consumption since the Second World War, and with it
has come a sizeable increase in degenerative diseases that affect
the circulatory system, joints, and muscles, and contribute significantly to the problem of cancer.

It is not yet clear exactly how eating red meat is linked to cancer. Possibly, acids in the gut turn amino acids in meat into carcinogenic nitrosamines. If transit time in the gut is slow due to a
low-fiber diet, these substances can cause damage to the cells in
the intestine wall as well as to other tissues once they are absorbed
into the blood. This mechanism is responsible for only a proportion
of bowel cancers, however. Ultimately, scientists may find that the
link between cancer and red meat can be traced to viruses that are
passed up the food chain. This could mean that the BSE crisis is
just the tip of the iceberg. It is striking that the 1998 findings of the
prospective study by Doctors Key and Thorogood showed that
vegetarians are 40 to 50 percent less likely to die of cancer than
meat eaters. This is an enormous difference, and it is urgent that

we discover the underlying mechanism behind this link. Meanwhile, it is vital to cut down consumption of red meat to a minimum or eliminate it altogether.

The British government's Committee on the Medical Aspects of Food advises a reduction of meat consumption in your daily diet to no more than 100 grams (around 3 ounces). This allowance includes the meat in products such as pasta sauces and pizza. It is far better, though, to avoid having meat every day, and if possible to eliminate it altogether from the diet. If you are especially fond of meat and unable to give it up completely, have a meat meal once a week, using only the best quality organic meat if possible. By doing this, you put quality before quantity and will really enjoy the occasional treat more, knowing that overall you are protecting yourself and your family by making this key dietary change.

Whenever you do eat meat, it is also important to eat vegetables or a salad along with it. The carcinogenic effects of meat are lessened by the presence in the digestive system of the vitamins and other plant chemicals in vegetables, and the fiber content of vegetables ensures a rapid transit time through the gut for the meat, another protective factor.

Be wary of simply replacing red meat with chicken or fish. While these are preferable forms of protein, excess consumption may still increase risk. Even more important, avoid replacing meat with cheese. All cheese is very high in animal fat; thus a diet of pizza or pasta covered in cheese sauce will make matters worse, not better. The best move for those who feel inspired to "go all the way" is to become completely vegan and eliminate animal products from the diet altogether. The major protein sources then become beans, lentils, nuts, and seeds, which provide the ideal balance of protein and healthy fats. Almost everyone who goes vegan says the improvement in their health, energy, and well-being is quite remarkable, and they wish they had done it years ago!

Animal Fats

Animal fats are major contributors to obesity, and they also appear to carry a risk of cancer in their own right. Therefore, as just mentioned, it is important not to swap meat for cheese and other high-fat dairy products. Keep their consumption to a bare minimum. Dramatically reduce your intake of cheese, butter, milk, and cream, and cut down on yogurt and eggs. Trim the fat off meat, give up cooking with animal fats such as lard and bacon grease, and keep the use of butter and cream in cooking to a minimum. Animal fats for cooking should be replaced with vegetable oils, and enriching recipes with butter and cream should be avoided, for this sort of food preparation is at the root of the Western dietary and obesity problem.

Certain fats are vital to our health; these are the essential fatty acids. The most helpful of these are omega-3 fatty acids, which are found in fish oils and linseed oil (flaxseed oil), as well as in many nuts and seeds. One way to ensure an adequate intake of these vital fatty acids is to take linseed-oil tablets or to sprinkle crushed or whole linseeds over other foods. Even with the healthier vegetable oils, like olive oil, it is important to avoid their excessive use in dressings and cooking. After all, these are still a type of fat, and their overconsumption will lead to obesity and all the associated health problems.

Foods That Include Preservatives and Additives

It is best to avoid all foods that have been pickled, smoked, salted, or preserved with additives such as sodium nitrate (saltpeter) and others. Saltpeter can combine with protein to promote the formation of carcinogenic nitrosamines in preserved foods such as sausages and salami. Smoking food can lead to the formation of carcinogenic polycyclic aromatic hydrocarbons. Sadly, this means that both bacon and sausage, two staple ingredients of the traditional American breakfast, must go—or at least become a very rare treat. In addition to the additives in sausages and the harmful substances in smoked bacon, the high animal-fat content of these foods and the superheating of their fats during cooking make them key items to avoid. We must all convert to delicious and healthy breakfasts of fresh fruit salads, cereals, oatmeal or whole-grain farina, pancakes or waffles, and whole-grain toast, and give up our addiction to fried breakfast foods.

The salting and pickling of food has been shown to produce higher levels of esophageal and stomach cancer in Japan and of nose and throat cancer in China; there is a serious need in both of these countries to exchange certain traditional dietary habits for healthy new ones.

In general, food additives should be avoided, as should artificial sweeteners, which have also been linked to cancer. Although food additives (along with other forms of environmental pollutants) have been shown to cause less than 1 percent of cancers, this should be enough to encourage us to eat whole foods that do not contain additives. The advice here is: Eat only fresh food, avoiding anything that is stored long term in jars or cans or that is "enhanced" or preserved in any artificial way.

In this day and age when fresh and frozen food is available in all seasons, there is no need for people to eat preserved foods— such as bright-green, mushy canned peas. Preserving food artificially or heightening its appeal with false colors or flavors is unnecessary, and such foods should be eliminated from the diet and replaced with (preferably organic) whole foods that are additive- and preservative-free.

COOKING METHODS THAT INCREASE CANCER RISK

Cooking methods that should be avoided to reduce the risk of cancer include:

- ❖ charbroiling and barbecuing
- ❖ frying, especially in superheated oils
- ❖ smoking
- ❖ microwaving (potentially)

Charbroiling and Barbecuing

As delicious as they may be, charbroiled or barbecued meats are definitely associated with increased cancer risk. The parts of meat that become charred contain dangerous polycyclic aromatic hydrocarbons that can cause DNA damage. Unfortunately, this means we should throw out our barbecue grills and restrain ourselves from ordering charbroiled foods in restaurants. Over the last ten years, home barbecuing has significantly increased in popularity; barbecue grills are now available in every hardware store and garden center; charcoal is sold at most supermarkets. Barbecues are associated with good times and a party atmosphere, and barbecued food is increasingly available at restaurants and outdoor events. Sadly, we must reverse this trend in order to help prevent cancer.

Advice in other health-related literature suggests that if people are going to eat barbecued or charbroiled food, they should first take vitamin C, beta-carotene, and other antioxidant vitamins and minerals to protect themselves. This may be a good idea, but it is much better to avoid these foods entirely. As with red meat, if you do eat charbroiled or barbecued food, it is vital to eat plenty of vegetables and salad along with it—not just the garnish of a solitary lettuce leaf and tomato slice that we so often see when eating out.

An added source of danger when barbecuing is the toxic lighter fluid that is usually poured over the charcoal. If meat is placed on the barbecue before the fuel has fully burned off, the fuel vapor can be absorbed into the meat's fat, which is then absorbed into our system when we eat the meat. It is therefore important to make sure any lighter fluid used is completely burned off before putting food on the barbecue; take special care if more fuel is added later in the cooking process.

Frying

Avoid frying as much as possible, because the high temperatures involved can break down fats into carcinogenic free radicals. It is particularly important to avoid heating cooking oils and fats until they smoke. In addition, the use of animal fats such as lard or bacon grease should definitely be avoided because of their high levels of saturated fats. Also avoid reusing old oil for deep-frying, as oil degenerates every time it is used. In fact, it is much better to abandon deep-frying and deep-fried foods altogether as they are extremely fattening and therefore convey risk for both cancer and heart disease. Safer ways of frying, such as stir-frying and water frying, are described in the section on healthy cooking methods, in Chapter 4.

Smoking

As with charbroiling and barbecuing, the smoking of food can cause dangerous changes to the proteins or fats in fish and meat. It is therefore wise to eliminate smoked foods from your diet to reduce the risk of cancer.

Microwaving

As yet, there is no direct evidence linking microwaved foods to an increased cancer risk. However, as explained in Chapter 1, microwaving heats food to a very high level, causing unnecessary destruction of vital nutrients and leaving food dangerously hot. If proper cooling times for microwaved foods are not observed, the excessive heat can damage the lining of the mouth, esophagus, and stomach. It is therefore inadvisable to use a microwave—because of its effect on the nutritional value of foods and because it breaks down the vitamins, plant enzymes, and phytochemicals that can protect against cancer. It is too soon to know for sure whether the use of a microwave is in itself safe, but certainly manufacturers' instructions must be followed to the letter. Ideally, we should eliminate the microwave oven from our lives and return to more traditional cooking methods.

SMOKING AND TOBACCO PRODUCTS

The message about smoking and cancer could not be clearer. Smoking of any sort—whether it is cigarette, pipe, or cigar smoking—should be stopped. It is also important to avoid smokeless tobacco products, such as chewing tobacco and snuff, as they are associated with cancer of the mouth, larynx, and esophagus and compound the risk of the alcohol-associated cancers.

In addition to giving up smoking yourself, it is vital to keep away from other people's smoke—at home, at work, or when socializing. Make it absolutely clear to friends and family that your home and car are nonsmoking areas. Campaign to make your place of work a smoke-free zone if humanly possible. Sit in nonsmoking areas of trains and public buildings, and always ask specifically to be seated in the nonsmoking section of restaurants. The more this is demanded, the greater the allocation of space for nonsmokers will be. If you are in charge at work or at any public place, take a stand and declare it a nonsmoking zone.

Most important is the need to be responsible around children. Never smoke in front of children or pregnant women or if you are pregnant yourself. It is completely wrong that the environment of a child, born or unborn, can be polluted in this way. Adults who smoke should never put children at increased risk of lung disease and cancer.

There is good news about the rates of death from lung cancer in the United States and Great Britain. Since 1970, the American lung-cancer death rate has reduced by half in middle-age men. In 1950, the UK had the worst lung-cancer death rates in the world but has seen the best decrease since. In 2000, Sir Richard Doll and Sir Richard Peto, from the Imperial Cancer Research Fund's Oxford unit, reported that, compared to Doll's 1950 results, widespread cessation of smoking in the UK had cut in half the number of lung cancer deaths. The study found that of men who continue to smoke, 16 percent will die before age seventy-five; but for those who stop before age fifty, the death rate goes down to 6 percent. For those who stop before age thirty, the death rate is less than 2 percent.

This good news compares starkly to the overall worldwide picture, however, because of the rise in lung-cancer deaths in developing countries. In the twentieth century, one hundred million tobacco deaths occurred worldwide. It is predicted that if smoking continues to increase at today's rates, one billion deaths from smoking will occur in the twenty-first century.

Giving Up Smoking

In developed countries everyone knows that smoking is dangerous, and yet many people continue to smoke. This is another example of how information alone does not change behavior. To quit smoking or using smokeless tobacco products, we must address both nicotine addiction and emotional dependency. While nicotine is admittedly very physically addictive, most people who smoke are as hooked emotionally as they are chemically.

Nicotine Addiction

Usually, after a person stops smoking, the withdrawal effects from nicotine last only a few days, and the chemical craving is likely to be gone within a week or two. If you feel you are chemically dependent on cigarettes, it is possible to get help from the use of nicotine patches, nicotine chewing gum, or even nicotine inhalers. These provide a substitute nicotine fix by which you can wean yourself off nicotine slowly, knowing that you are protected meanwhile from the carcinogens in the tobacco smoke. Quitting smoking this way, however, just puts off the "evil hour" when you must break the link and give up the nicotine dependency entirely.

Emotional Dependency

Ultimately, success in quitting smoking almost invariably revolves around being sufficiently motivated and having the right level of support emotionally. So it is in these areas that we should focus our greatest efforts.

Most smokers smoke because it helps them control difficult feelings, such as anxiety, nervousness, self-consciousness, upset, loneliness, anger, or grief. Nicotine is a stimulant that gives people a slight lift. The physiological changes brought about by tobacco use temporarily change people's state of mind, to some extent blotting out the feelings they had before they picked up a cigarette, pipe, cigar, or smokeless product. The problem is that the lift is only temporary, and the harmful effects often leave people feeling more irritable or anxious than they were before. As with all drugs, the simplest solution seems to be to have more, and so the vicious cycle continues.

Because of the underlying emotional reasons why people smoke, it is ridiculous to think that either good advice or scaring people with medical data will make a big difference in their habit. The increasing number of therapeutic and self-help smoking-cessation programs in the community, both private and nonprofit, means more people than ever now have a chance to understand their underlying state of mind. Improving our state of mind and emotions depends on:

❖ allowing yourself to recognize, feel, and express emotions

❖ learning to make your needs known clearly and ask for what you need

❖ developing loving relationships so you will feel safe and secure

❖ developing a loving and nurturing relationship with yourself

❖ developing inner strength and calmness by the use of self-help techniques such as relaxation, meditation, visualization, yoga, and tai chi

❖ developing outlets for your creativity and self-expression

Changing our underlying psychological problems quite often requires some "emotional reeducation." People who need to smoke to suppress their emotions are likely to have grown up in environments where it was unsafe or embarrassing to express how they felt. They require support and encouragement and sometimes permission in order to admit and express their feelings. It is hard to change emotional habits or patterns on our own, and it may well take a dozen or more sessions with a counselor to experience a different way of dealing with feelings. Counseling is particularly helpful if you time it so that you have a couple of sessions before giving up smoking, and then continue during the crucial period when you are first coming off cigarettes, when emotions that smoking has suppressed for a long time begin to surface.

In a good counseling relationship, people are able to let go and express their feelings, learn how to deal with emotions differently, develop a new nurturing relationship with themselves, and develop a positive relationship with the counselor on which they can model other good relationships in the future. They are also able to explore the whole question of expressing themselves fully and achieving their potential in life. In this situation, people learn how to communicate well and how to explore and define their needs, but sometimes they need to take the process farther by seeking out assertiveness training. If you are too shy or embarrassed to voice your feelings and needs, often find yourself bullied or overwhelmed, and resort to smoking to calm yourself, assertiveness training may be a very good idea. You will be trained in techniques that 1) will help you identify what you are feeling and needing and 2) will teach you to express your needs clearly and repeatedly until they are met. As well as being able to control the frustration and hurt that result from continually being trampled on, you will gain additional benefits by learning these techniques.

Another way to get help is to join a support group, where you will have the opportunity to talk about how you feel. Because these groups offer less one-on-one support than individual therapy, they may not be direct enough for some people. Finally, the American Lung Association offers a Freedom from Smoking program (see the Resources section).

Relaxation Techniques

Some relaxation methods were mentioned in the section on emotional dependency on food. Nonetheless, it is worth reemphasizing that by practicing yoga, yoga breathing, tai chi, relaxation, and meditation, and doing other sorts of physical exercise can make an enormous difference in your state of mind. Relaxation is like changing the idling speed on a car. When a car engine turns over too quickly, it wastes precious fuel and puts strain on the engine. To solve this problem, a mechanic can reset the idling speed at a much lower level. Similarly, when stress, worry, and perpetual hurry speed us up too much, making us tense, irritable, and inefficient, we can use relaxation techniques to attain a calmer, gentler state of being.

As with changing the way we deal with our emotions, it can be difficult to learn to relax on our own. It may be necessary at first to be relaxed passively by someone else. You can achieve this through a massage, aromatherapy, or reflexology session, or by going for spiritual healing. (For more about spiritual healing, see Chapter 4.) Once you begin to experience what it is like to feel relaxed, you can build upon this at home with the use of relaxation tapes or CDs or by learning relaxation techniques from a relaxation therapist. An alternative is to attend relaxation, yoga, or tai chi classes. The beauty of yoga and tai chi, both of which come from the East, is that they combine physical exercise with relaxation, breathing, and meditation exercises, and thus are specifically designed to simultaneously strengthen the body while calming the mind and nervous system. This is exactly what is needed for most smokers, whose nervous systems get progressively more jangled as they continue to smoke. (Achieving optimal physical and mental health will be dealt with fully in Chapter 4, and contacts for counseling, relaxation, yoga, tai chi, and meditation classes can be found in the Resources section at the back of the book.)

Social Aspects of Smoking

Another aspect of giving up smoking involves breaking the established smoking pattern—the reflex action of smoking at the end of meals, when drinking alcohol (either at home or in bars and restaurants), after a difficult day on the job, or at certain routine times during your day (such as during your break at work). To overcome these habits, you must first identify what triggers them and then try to form a strategy to change your behavior at these key moments.

For most smokers, the most common trigger point is the end of a meal. Try to find something else to do at this and other trigger points to replace having a cigarette. For example, if you are at home you could lie down and listen to a ten-minute relaxation tape. You could go outside and get some fresh air in the garden or take a walk around the block. It may be a good time to read or even take a nap. At work you also have to be creative, although it may still be possible to sit quietly for a few minutes and do a relaxation exercise—even if it is in the bathroom!

If your trigger point is when drinking alcohol at social or business meetings, finding replacement tactics is obviously much harder. Indeed, this is usually the time when people's good resolutions crumble and those who have successfully given up for a few days lapse into smoking again. If socializing is a vulnerable situation for you, then it may be wise to avoid drinking alcohol and your usual social meetings while you are giving up smoking. It may even be a good idea to avoid going to restaurants, bars, and clubs, where you know you will be severely tempted, until you have stopped smoking altogether for around six weeks.

Quite often, newly reformed nonsmokers find smoky atmospheres difficult to cope with. This is because the cleansing mechanisms in their lungs and windpipe are coming back to life, and the irritation, unpleasant taste, and smell of smoke are now really noticeable and hard to take. It is a good sign when this starts to happen; it shows that the body is beginning to recover from smoking. It may also serve to strengthen your resolve to give up the use of tobacco for good.

In terms of secondhand smoke, bars and clubs are the worst places to be. Large crowds of smokers are often crowded together in a very confined space, often with grossly inadequate ventilation. Secondhand smoke is classified as an occupational cancer risk for bar employees, and there is a desperate need in society for nonsmoking bars and clubs. Try to avoid smoky places if you can, or complain regularly and vociferously to the owners or even to the local regulatory agencies if you think a health risk is being caused by inadequate ventilation.

Therapeutic Help

Many people find hypnosis or self-hypnosis useful in helping them overcome tobacco cravings or reflex-action smoking in response to key triggers. The hypnotist enables smokers to break their smoking patterns by replacing that self-destructive behavior with positive thoughts and feelings. Another therapeutic technique that has proven effective is acupuncture. The acupuncturist manipulates certain pressure points of the body to liberate chemicals called *endorphins*—neuropeptides in the brain that impart a feeling of satisfaction and thus help to reduce the urge to smoke.

A practice that promotes relaxation especially during the first six weeks of quitting smoking is having regular weekly or twice-weekly massages. Given the current high cost of cigarettes, the expense of regular massages is probably less or at least equal to the money you now spend on cigarettes.

It is also helpful while giving up tobacco to take:

❖ 1,000 mg of vitamin C three times per day

❖ 50 mg of B complex per day

❖ 100 mg of zinc orotate per day

These vitamins and minerals:

❖ help repair lung-tissue damage caused by long-term smoking (particularly the zinc orotate);

❖ boost the immune system and protect against infections (particularly vitamin C). When smoking stops, the lungs temporarily start to secrete more mucus. This can make people prone to infections such as bronchitis or even pneumonia;

❖ help calm the nervous system (particularly vitamin B).

But even with the support of all the approaches mentioned above, the most important thing is having the *intention* to stop.

Forming the Intention to Stop Smoking

It may sound obvious, but the more you want to stop smoking, the easier it will be and the more likely you are to succeed. So if you are a smoker, take time right now to think about how important it is to stop smoking.

Write the answers to the following questions:

- ❖ Why do you want to give up smoking?

- ❖ What do you get from smoking?

- ❖ What will make it difficult for you to give up smoking?

- ❖ How can you replace the benefits you get from smoking in a healthy way?

- ❖ How chemically dependent are you on cigarettes?

- ❖ Will you require help in the form of nicotine replacement to stop?

- ❖ How emotionally dependent are you on cigarettes?

- ❖ What level of emotional support will you need to give up smoking?

- ❖ What could you do instead of smoking at your normal "trigger points" to avoid having a cigarette?

Look at your answers. Are you really ready to give up smoking? Once you have decided that you are ready to commit yourself to quitting smoking, take a fresh piece of paper and write in large letters a clear statement of intention: "I choose to give up smoking now" or "I now give up smoking" or "I successfully give up smoking now"—whatever form feels the most comfortable to you.

Then write out a second statement, listing all the support you will need—for example, a counselor, relaxation therapist, hypnotherapist, acupuncturist, massage therapist, support group, a "stop-smoking" agency or clinic, a doctor, nicotine patches, etc.

Third, write down the people you will ask to support you in giving up smoking. It is important to consciously enroll partners, key family members, colleagues, and friends in case the going gets tough during the first few weeks. Tell them your intention so they are witnesses to your commitment. Explain exactly the type of help you will need, and how they may best support you. This may be anything from asking them to avoid smoking in front of you, offering you cigarettes, or confronting you with problems during the first six weeks, to asking them to be extra kind and patient with you. Or you can simply explain that you will not be socializing as normal until you have beaten the habit. You may also wish to tell them how you want them to react if they see you smoking!

Next, until you are well and truly clear of your smoking habit, repeat your commitment to yourself—out loud is good—every single day. You may want to post your written intention in a prominent place in the house or at work, but actually saying it to yourself each day and visualizing yourself as a nonsmoker are very powerful practices. As a reward to yourself for your day-by-day success, you could save the money you would normally spend on cigarettes and use it to buy something for your closet or home, or for a lovely vacation or some other treat.

In summary, the importance of giving up smoking cannot be stressed enough. The benefits will have repercussions in every area of your life. Best of all, you will feel much better, happier, and fitter within just a few weeks of stopping.

ALCOHOL

When Angela Burns was diagnosed with breast cancer, it forced her to reevaluate her life. She was a manager with a large international retail organization, and liked to work hard and play hard. She is the first to admit that this meant drinking heavily on a regular basis. Angela was first diagnosed with breast cancer in 1991, when a mammogram picked up an early tumor. She underwent a lumpectomy and radiation and went back to work and her old lifestyle without a second thought.

Only when she was diagnosed in 1995 with a second lump in the same breast, for which she needed a mastectomy, did Angela realize that she needed to start thinking about making some serious changes in her life. During rest and recuperation after the operation, she became aware for the first time in her working life of just how tired she was. She also had huge regrets about not taking action after the first diagnosis.

A doctor suggested she look at what the Bristol Cancer Help Centre offered, and Angela joined the residential week-long course. Since then, Angela has made lots of life changes. Psychologically, she discovered she was not taking care of herself properly and always put her team at work and other members of her family before herself. Energy-wise, she had run her batteries completely down because of her fast lifestyle. Despite her doubts about spiritual healing, she tried it, and now finds it both wonderfully calming and energizing. She also uses reflexology and relaxation techniques.

Angela stopped drinking alcohol every day, enjoying a drink only on the weekends, and cut out hard liquor completely. She switched to goat's cheese and sheep's cheese initially, but has now cut dairy products out of her diet altogether. She eats a little fish and chicken but has stopped eating salt, smoked foods, red meat, and pre-prepared foods like pâtés and pork pies, and doesn't drink coffee. Angela is now on a low-fat diet, eating organic fruit and vegetables whenever possible. All this doesn't mean she has become completely puritanical. She does indulge in fish and chips and a pint of beer every now and again!

The biggest change was that Angela decided to reduce her stress dramatically and relinquish her demanding job, retiring at the age of fifty. Doing this meant it was far easier to seriously reduce her intake of alcohol once she no longer "needed" it to manage her stress. She now works part-time at an enjoyable variety of paid and volunteer work mixed with plenty of gentle, fun, creative projects. Five years after the secondary diagnosis she feels fine and looks radiant. Her new motto is to enjoy all things in moderation, and her new game plan is to drink one bottle of good champagne a week rather than seven bottles of the cheap stuff!

Changing Your Use of Alcohol

Two units of alcohol a day for women and three for men are the maximum recommended safe levels. One unit of alcohol is equal to 6 fluid ounces of wine, 8 ounces (half a pint) of beer, or 1 ounce of liquor. Women who regularly consume 3 units a day and men who drink 4 units daily incur progressive risk to their health, including an increased risk of cancer. Alcohol increases the risk of cancers of the mouth, throat, larynx (voice box), esophagus (gullet), liver, and breast, and the risk goes up as consumption increases. People who smoke as well as drink alcohol over the safe limit are at a considerably higher risk.

Even when staying within the recommended daily amounts, there is a good chance a person can become dependent on alcohol. As with smoking, alcohol dependence can be both chemical and emotional. If you have become fixed in a pattern of regular drinking or actively need a drink at specific times of the day or during social situations, it is time to look seriously at why you are dependent on alcohol and to start to find healthier ways to meet the needs you currently fulfill with a drink.

Alcohol and its by-products are very toxic to the body, causing premature aging, gut and liver disease, diseases of the nervous system, and cardiovascular problems. Heavy drinking increases the risk of certain cancers and can cause social and emotional distress. Alcohol, smoking, and stress are currently the biggest thieves of vitality and health in Western society. Of course, these things go hand in hand, since stress increases our urge to drink and to smoke.

Ideally, it is best to stop drinking alcohol on a daily basis altogether. You should allow at least two to three days after an intake of alcohol before drinking again in order to give the body a chance to detoxify and heal itself. People who drink regularly get used to the effects of alcohol and are less sensitive to its toxicity. But as anybody who drinks intermittently knows, it takes at least two days to feel fully recovered after an evening of drinking three or more units of alcohol. Try to make alcohol something just for special times, and think twice before routinely having a drink at social gatherings, business lunches, or when you get home from work.

Chemical Dependency

If you are hooked on alcohol and need a drink to stop feeling bad physically—to stop shaking or feeling sick—you may need medical help to wean yourself off it. Medication is available that is much less addictive than alcohol and helps to calm the mind while the body gets used to alcohol withdrawal. Unlike nicotine replacement therapy, this medicine cannot be bought over the counter; it requires a doctor's or psychiatrist's prescription. Because long-term heavy drinking can leave you feeling pretty roughed-up physically and psychologically, you may even need to spend a few days in a hospital or treatment center to help you through the withdrawal period. However, once through this difficult time, you will start to feel better than you have for ages. Ask yourself, "Am I sick and tired of feeling sick and tired?" and resolve to become free of alcohol dependence. Alcohol is a seriously nasty drug, and the sooner you can get off it the better.

Emotional Dependency

As with cigarettes, many people have an emotional dependence on alcohol. Although they use alcohol to cover up feelings of anxiety, insecurity, and poor self-esteem, its regular use in fact deteriorates a person's mental state. People who drink excessive amounts of alcohol tend to be aggressive and violent and to suffer heightened feelings of guilt and remorse. In general, thinking processes are slowed down, and with continued heavy use the damage to the nervous system can be catastrophic, with severe memory loss and impaired sensation and muscle function in the limbs.

Because excessive alcohol consumption causes such a vicious cycle of psychological problems, after a long period of alcohol abuse it is often an enormous task to rebuild emotional health and gain a strong positive self-image. Once you recognize any of the signs of alcohol dependency in yourself, it is important to tackle these problems before you find yourself dealing with full-blown alcoholism. If you think you are an alcoholic, or seriously alcohol dependent, the most effective and best known means of getting support is through Alcoholics Anonymous. Their famous and very effective twelve-step program helps people to let go of alcohol and thus free themselves from the behavior and attitudes that accompany their drinking, replacing them with healthier coping strategies. If your drinking is not heavy enough to merit this level of intervention but you realize that you are somewhat psychologically dependent on alcohol, then it would be wise to follow the advice given earlier for giving up smoking: go to a counselor, join a support group, and learn to develop inner strength through the use of complementary therapies and self-help techniques. You will then be able to develop healthier ways of getting your emotional needs met.

What makes alcohol so popular is its power to relax and to loosen inhibitions. In the early stages of intoxication, people feel a lift in their emotional state. But this turns into a depressant effect after about 3 units. Instead of relying on alcohol for these effects, you can learn how to achieve a deep state of relaxation naturally through relaxation and meditation techniques. Once you master these techniques you can use them whenever you would normally reach for a drink. When you first get home from work is a good time to employ such a technique, because often that one drink to relax you turns into two, three, or more. The result is probably a very nonproductive, uncreative evening, one that leaves you hungover and less able to function well the next day.

By contrast, half an hour of relaxation or meditation allows the tension and exhaustion of the day to melt away, leaving you refreshed, open, and receptive, and able to enjoy a more constructive and creative time. Indeed, people who meditate regularly become progressively calmer, and their desire for alcohol diminishes greatly. Once a meditation technique is established, alcohol becomes less and less desirable anyway, because the states of mind reached through meditation are so much more pleasant and exciting than those reached with alcohol.

If you need alcohol because you feel shy on a date or before getting intimate with your partner, again, it is far, far better to learn to relax and develop communication skills than to use drink as a social lubricant. Once you get to know a new partner, loosening up together by using relaxation techniques and massage with soothing oils in candlelight will result in a much more pleasurable and richer experience than if you were both drunk! As for the lift given by alcohol, it is very brief and is quickly replaced with a depression of all the senses. There are many other ways of becoming excited and happier that do not involve feeling sick and ill the next day! If you rely on alcohol to get you through social situations, you may well need counseling or assertiveness training to help build your confidence. Another option is a massage course to build up your physical confidence and develop new ways of breaking the ice with a new partner.

The Social Side of Alcohol

Many people automatically pick up a drink in response to social cues, irrespective of whether they have any actual desire for one. Also, within some families or segments of society, people are hardwired from a young age to feel that unless they get drunk they have not had a good time. Drinking may even become competitive in some social circles, with people trying to outdo each other in terms of alcohol consumption. Others with a more compulsive personality just keep drinking—in the same way that some people just keep eating—whether they really want to or not. For all these reasons and many more, we in general drink far too much alcohol in unthinking, indiscriminate ways. Therefore, it is vital for our health to think about how we want to drink and to get back in control of our drinking habits.

Without doubt, nothing compares to an exquisite bottle of wine to accompany a good meal, a beautiful bottle of champagne to celebrate a special occasion, or a glass of really cold beer on a hot summer day. These are some of the great pleasures of life. The advice is the same as that given for red meat: replace quantity with quality. Drink smaller quantities of excellent (preferably organic) alcohol at special times, rather than large quantities of inferior alcohol all the time as a socially acceptable form of Valium!

To develop new drinking habits, it may be wise, as when stopping smoking, to change your normal social routine, avoiding the bars or clubs you usually visit until you have reoriented yourself. You may need to take this even further if it proves impossible to go back to those places without overdrinking. If this is the case, you may need to consider a more radical change, replacing evenings normally spent in a bar with things like exercise, classes, or creative self-expressive projects that will probably bring you greater satisfaction in the long run. You could also spend this time getting closer to those you love or taking time to be by yourself.

There is of course the theory that a glass of wine a day protects against coronary heart disease and heart attacks. This protection is probably due to two factors. First, plant nutrients in grapes include important vitamins, minerals, enzymes, and other phytochemicals. Second, alcohol has a relaxing effect. Both of these effects, however, can be achieved in nontoxic ways—the first, by eating fruits and vegetables, including grapes; the second, by learning and practicing relaxation. Overall, it must surely be better to avoid the toxic effects of alcohol and to get the benefits in safe, healthy ways through diet and relaxation.

If more and more adults change their drinking habits, a new attitude toward alcohol will pass down through the generations and we will begin to see a reduction in the terrible suffering caused by excessive use of this very toxic drug.

In summary, healthy use of alcohol means:

❖ avoiding drinking alcohol every day

❖ drinking no more than 3 units for women and 4 units for men at any one time

❖ recognizing and meeting emotional needs in healthy ways rather than by using alcohol

❖ seeking medical and psychological help if addicted to alcohol

HORMONE REPLACEMENT THERAPY AND THE PILL

Hormone Replacement Therapy (HRT)

The conventional medical opinion is that the risks of hormone replacement therapy are outweighed by its protective effects, such as preventing osteoporosis. However, knowing that many cancers, particularly breast cancers, are hormonally sensitive makes me extremely worried about the use of HRT. My own advice is to avoid taking estrogen-based or estrogen-progesterone combined HRT altogether unless there is a medical reason (such as osteoporosis) to do so. If vaginal soreness or dryness is a problem after menopause, you can use estrogen cream or pessaries, which can be obtained from your doctor. Where a low bone density has been diagnosed and osteoporosis seems likely, or there is a strong family history of osteoporosis, it is up to each individual to make an informed choice based on her own circumstances and age.

Progesterone HRT

A new trend is to give progesterone-only HRT, which is considered a safer option. This is because progesterone is thought to be a less stimulatory hormone than estrogen. However, because some breast tumors are also progesterone-receptor positive, it would seem unwise at present to prescribe progesterone-only HRT on a wide scale until more is understood. My advice therefore is to avoid taking HRT altogether, relying on a healthy and fulfilling lifestyle with good diet and exercise to maintain health and beauty after menopause.

The skin of the body can be kept beautiful with oils and body creams, as can the skin of the face. Taking regular vitamin E and flaxseed oils, and using facial creams containing retin-A will also help keep the face looking good. Hot flashes are helped by vitamin E and flaxseed oil, and herbal preparations such as agnus castus, black cohosh, and Menopausal Herb Formula (see the Resources section) can help to smooth a woman's passage through menopause. Many women find that reflexology helps to ease the hormonal transition, because both the pituitary gland and the ovaries can be stimulated through reflexes in the feet.

The Pill

Advice on oral contraceptives in relation to cancer is harder. The conventional medical view is that the benefits outweigh the risks because the risks of the Pill stop when a woman goes off it; and because in general the Pill is taken by women under the age of forty-five, in whom the risk of breast cancer is much lower. This is all very well, but increasing numbers of young women are getting breast cancer, and the disease is often more virulent because of the high levels of circulating estrogen. It is therefore better for women to use an alternative to the Pill as soon as other forms of contraception are suitable for them. During the early years of sexual activity, however, the benefits of the Pill still probably outweigh the risks. Thereafter, it would be much better to use barrier methods such as the diaphragm, condoms, or an intrauterine device (IUD). Generally, an IUD is only recommended for women who have had children. Additionally, the IUD and the diaphragm do not protect against infectious diseases that can cause AIDS and cervical cancer. So unless you are in a monogamous relationship with someone who has been confirmed infection free, condom use is vital.

INFECTIONS

The main hope of preventing cancer is by controlling infections such as HPV (human papillomavirus) and HIV, the three hepatitis viruses (A, B, and C), herpes simplex, and the viruses in Africa that cause lymphomas (which are linked with malarial disease). Prevention of HPV, HIV, and hepatitis can be achieved by engaging in safe sex, by absolutely avoiding the use of intravenous recreational drugs (all these blood-borne diseases can be spread via contaminated needles), and by following other health practices that reduce exposure to the blood of possible carriers. It is important for everyone to maintain good sexual hygiene with new partners; it is even more important for those practicing anal sex, where the likelihood of trauma and infection through blood contact is higher.

For those who know they are carrying these viruses, absolute integrity in terms of their sexual practice is essential; they need to inform all potential partners of their health status. This will allow new partners to make informed choices about what sorts of sexual activity they wish to get involved in before putting themselves at risk.

Work is continuing on vaccinations against all these viruses, and it is likely that within our lifetimes such vaccines will be developed to protect people who are vulnerable. Vaccinations are already available against hepatitis A and B, and in some developing countries, where these viruses are more prevalent, vaccination programs are now under way. Consider being vaccinated against hepatitis A and/or B if you believe yourself to be at risk, either through travel or because you have an infected partner.

SUNLIGHT

For years, deeply tanned skin has been considered the pinnacle of health, beauty, and sexiness. Now cancer researchers tell us there is no such thing as a safe and healthy tan. It was estimated that more than eight hundred thousand Americans would be diagnosed with skin cancer in 2001. In fact, in the United States, the occurrence of melanoma, an often untreatable and deadly form of skin cancer, is rising faster than that of any other cancer.

We all crave sunshine and, indeed, become ill without it. We need sunshine on our skin to create vitamin D, which keeps our bones healthy. Without enough sunlight, we can also develop seasonal affective disorder (SAD), which is a form of depression. However, in order to stay safe in the sun the advice is:

- Avoid exposing your skin between 11:00 A.M. and 3:00 P.M. (or 10:00 A.M. to 4:00 P.M. if you live in the South).

- Cover your skin with loose cotton clothes, a sun hat, and sunglasses.

- Take care not to burn your skin, being particularly careful if there is a cool breeze or light cloud cover.

- Wear a sunscreen that offers an SPF of at least fifteen (see below) as well as broad-spectrum protection (that is, protection from both UVA and UVB rays).

- Protect yourself when swimming; you can get sunburned in the water.

❖ Pay attention to the solar UV index in television, Internet, and radio weather forecasts at home and abroad.

❖ Be extra sure to protect children, and keep babies under twelve months out of the sun completely.

❖ Take special care if you have fair skin, blonde or red hair, and freckles, because your type of skin burns more easily than most.

Don't make the mistake of thinking you have nothing to worry about if you only go out in the sun for two weeks on vacation. It is even more important to protect yourself if you get a rare sudden burst of intense sunshine. It is also untrue that a tan from a tanning bed will prepare you for tanning in the sun. Tanning beds are based on UVA light rather than UVB light, which is the light in the sun's rays that burns the skin (sunlight contains both UVA and UVB light). People with dark skin do not burn as easily as those with fair skin; nonetheless, black and Asian people can also get sunburned.

The SPF (sun protection factor) listed on a bottle of sunscreen indicates how long you can stay in the sun without burning. For example, if you normally burn in ten minutes, wearing an SPF of fifteen will protect you fifteen times longer—that is, for two-and-a-half hours. But be aware: After two-and-a-half hours, no additional amount of sunscreen will stop you from burning. Avoid the common mistake of applying sunscreen too thinly; also, many are easily rubbed or washed off. Look for "sport" sunscreens, which are designed to avoid being washed off by perspiration or water. They also have a light, nongreasy consistency that some people prefer. Also, please note that during the two-and-a-half-hour period of coverage, it is necessary to regularly reapply sunscreen to ensure its effectiveness. Thereafter, it is essential to cover up with loose clothing and a sun hat or to sit in the shade. Some people worry about whether they will get sunburned through glass. This is unlikely, but it is possible to be exposed to some UVA rays, as they can pass through glass. You are most at risk if you have:

* a tendency to burn easily and tan only with difficulty

* had skin cancer

* a large number of moles

* sun spots or age spots, which are a warning sign that the skin has endured too much exposure to the sun and is more prone to skin cancer

It is recommended that you avoid tanning beds. These work mainly by pelting the skin with UVA radiation, which, though it doesn't burn the skin, is thought to play a potential role in the development of skin cancer. If you long for a tanned look, it is much safer to use self-tanning creams to achieve it.

ELECTROMAGNETIC RADIATION

The most common sources of concern about electromagnetic radiation in everyday life are mobile phones, microwave ovens, computers, electrical towers, and office environments where strong electromagnetic fields may be set up by large amounts of electrical and electronic equipment.

Mobile Phones

The advice is to keep use of mobile phones to a minimum and to use those with ear- and mouthpiece attachments (hands-free sets), rather than those that must be held to the head. Mobile phones can be kept in protective casing, and devices that keep emissions to an absolute minimum are now available (see the Resources section).

Microwave Ovens

As this book has already discussed, the use of microwave ovens should ideally be avoided. If you do use a microwave, follow the instructions to the letter, strictly observing cooling times for food. Make sure you do not use old or faulty equipment that may leak microwaves into the kitchen.

Computers

Always use a protective screen in front of your computer terminal to protect yourself against radiation. Take regular breaks from computer work. Do not leave your computer on if it is not in use. Try to avoid occupations that involve sitting in front of a computer all day every day.

Electricity

Living (or keeping animals) close to electrical towers is inadvisable because these structures emit strong electrical fields and positive ions that attract radioactive particles. It is also unhealthy to live over heavy-duty electrical cabling or near large electrical terminal points. Working in electric power stations may also be risky.

At work, it is up to your employer to ensure that exposure levels are safe. If you are concerned, ask your employer to have the levels checked. Of particular concern both at work and at home are extra-low-frequency electromagnetic fields, which have been specifically associated with cancer. Keep electrical equipment turned off when not in use, and do not sleep with an electric blanket switched on. If you have concerns about the levels of electromagnetic radiation around your home or place of work, seek advice from your electric utility, or consult with an environmental-testing lab.

Radioactivity

Naturally occurring radioactivity is linked to the presence of radon gas. The U.S. surgeon general has cited radon as the second-leading cause of lung cancer. The Environmental Protection Agency and the surgeon general recommend that all homes below the third floor and all schools be checked for radon. State environmental agencies can advise you about radon levels in your area and about how to have your home checked for radon (see the Resources section). In addition, if you live close to either a nuclear power station or a radioactive dumping site, it is advisable to check your home for background radiation levels. The more the public takes an interest in these matters, ultimately the safer we all will be.

If you work around radioactive materials, be extremely careful with their use and wear full protective clothing at all times.

Earth Energies

Knowing what electromagnetic fields and currents (sometimes known as earth energies) are affecting your property and how best to position beds and other furniture to minimize the negative effects of these energies is very interesting and advisable. If you are considering building a house or buying property, get the plot assessed first so that you can build in or buy an optimum location.

ENVIRONMENTAL POLLUTION

Carcinogens in the Home

It is important to try to eliminate all carcinogenic chemicals from the home environment. If at all possible, declare your home a non-smoking area. Refer to the list in Appendix 2 of all the household products that may contain carcinogens, and see if you can avoid their use. To learn which brands contain the offending chemicals, obtain a copy of *The Safe Shopper's Bible*. You can then select brands that are completely carcinogen free.

Occupational Carcinogens

Chemical Carcinogens

It is vital to ensure that you are not exposed to chemical carcinogens at work. Check the table of occupational hazards in Appendix 3, and check with the appropriate department at work to ensure that you are being adequately protected. All places where dangerous chemicals are used should have proper safety measures in place, including the wearing of protective clothing and the use of protective handling equipment. As mentioned earlier, if you are self-employed and using dangerous chemicals (for example, farmers, artists, and those in the building trades) you must be just as rigorous about safety measures as those working in a more closely monitored industrial environment.

Radiation

If you work as a radiologist or radiographer, or in any of the nuclear-fuel or power industries, it is vital to keep an accurate check of your levels of radiation exposure.

MEDICAL CAUSES

There are many medical causes of cancer (discussed in Chapter 1). These usually stem from the use of diagnostic electromagnetic radiation or from medicines and procedures used to treat medical conditions. To lower your risks, make sure medical testing is kept to a minimum. When accepting medical treatments of any sort, ask the doctor to advise you of all the side effects, so that you can make a properly informed choice about whether you wish to take the risks involved.

3

❖

Early Detection of Cancer

The seriousness of a cancer diagnosis may be greatly reduced if it is made early. It is therefore advisable to know the early warning symptoms of cancer. Become educated about how to check yourself and how to get the necessary medical screening.

INVESTIGATING EARLY SYMPTOMS

Symptoms to look out for that could indicate cancer include:

- ❖ a new or unusual lump anywhere on the body or in the abdomen
- ❖ a change in the appearance of a mole, or a sore on the skin or in the mouth that won't heal
- ❖ persistent coughing, hoarseness, or blood in the sputum
- ❖ prolonged constipation, diarrhea, or blood in the stool
- ❖ difficulty passing urine or blood in the urine
- ❖ unexplained weight loss
- ❖ unexplained fatigue
- ❖ difficulty swallowing and unexplained nausea

❖ severe headaches and odd neurological symptoms (i.e., malfunctions in the nervous system such as weakness or numbness)

❖ unexplained abdominal swelling

❖ vaginal bleeding between periods, and any vaginal bleeding after menopause

All these symptoms can result from conditions much less serious than cancer, and more often than not the doctor will reassure you that nothing is seriously wrong. However, it is important not to be reassured too quickly, until all the appropriate tests are done. All too often, physicians give reassurance on the basis of a clinical examination in the office, only to be proved wrong at a later date. Doctors expect patients to come back if symptoms persist, so it is very important to trust yourself and keep going back if you think something is not right. Far too many people visit their family doctor over and over again before they are sent for appropriate X rays, blood tests, or other investigations, only to discover that a cancer that could have been treated easily as a primary has now developed secondary spread. If you are concerned that your physician is not responding appropriately, get a second opinion from another doctor.

Lumps and Bumps

The usual medical response to the presentation of an unusual lump or bump is to biopsy it in order to make a histological diagnosis of the tissue within the lesion. This involves taking a sample of the lump with a needle or cutting a little bit of the lump out and sending it to a laboratory to be looked at under the microscope. A biopsy lets doctors know whether or not the lump is a cancer and if they need to look for other areas of disease within the body. Some controversy surrounds the practice of doing biopsies. If possible, it is better to have a lump removed altogether than to have it biopsied, because if the lump is cancerous there is a risk that cancer cells will spread along the track of the biopsy needle or the line of the incision. While it is more trouble for a doctor to remove a lump in its entirety, this procedure is safer, if it can be arranged.

The other option is to have an ultrasound, a CAT scan, or an MRI scan. These tests are often used anyway if the lump is deep within the body, and today, with the very high-level diagnostic skills available, it is often possible to diagnose cancer in these far less invasive ways.

So, if a lump of any sort appears on or underneath the skin, ask for it to be completely removed for analysis. If a lump appears in the breast, ask for it to be investigated first with ultrasound and/or mammography rather than a biopsy. If suspicion is high that it is cancerous, it is wise to proceed straight to a lumpectomy. This means removing the entire lump, including enough healthy breast tissue to be sure that the lump has been taken cleanly from the breast.

Lumps or bumps in the abdomen are also investigated by scans or ultrasound. Again, if suspicion is high, these can be removed either during a laparoscopy, where a tiny keyhole incision is made in the abdomen, or, if more serious, during investigative abdominal surgery.

Changes to the Skin and Mouth

If changes to the skin develop, you should see a dermatologist (skin specialist). Sores in the mouth that will not heal need the attention of either an oral surgeon or an ear, nose, and throat (ENT) surgeon. Again, if it is possible to avoid a biopsy and move straight to complete excision of the lesion, this is preferable. Usually, dermatologists, oral surgeons, and ENT specialists can tell by looking at these conditions whether they are cancerous, and are likely to go straight to excision instead of biopsy.

Coughing, Hoarseness, and Blood in the Sputum

This is one of the areas in which a cancer is easily missed. Many people suffer each year from colds, coughs, and chronic lung diseases such as bronchitis, bronchiectasis, and occupational lung disease, and most of us will have a sore throat at least once a year.

Usually, smokers have some soreness and hoarseness in the throat area all the time, so it is understandable that doctors do not send everyone with these symptoms for scans and X rays.

Persistent blood in the sputum, however, should definitely be taken seriously by doctors. Sometimes a sudden show of blood in the sputum that never reappears is caused by the rupturing of a small blood vessel in the lungs during heavy coughing. But if bleeding continues, it is likely to be from an area of ulceration in the windpipe (bronchus) or lungs, which could easily be due to cancer. People with persistent hoarseness should be sent to an ENT specialist. Blood in the sputum should be checked out with a bronchoscopy investigation. This involves a doctor looking directly at the windpipe and lungs, while the patient is under sedation, to see if there are any growths or areas of ulceration.

Persistent coughing merits a chest X ray and sputum test, and may also require a bronchoscopy. A sputum test can identify not only cancer cells, but also infectious agents and the presence of blood. Sputum samples are sent to three different parts of the pathology department, so if you are concerned, ask your doctor whether the sputum has been checked specifically for cancer cells.

Change in Bowel Habit

Again, this is a very difficult area for doctors to assess, as constipation, diarrhea, and even blood in the stool are very common. The most common cause of blood in the stool is hemorrhoids, which is caused by prolonged tightness of the anal sphincter muscle. Another explanation is anal fissures or fistulas, which are cracks in the skin of the anus. When you have hemorrhoids, fissures, or fistulas, you tend to know all about them because they make passing a stool very painful. People are likely to know, therefore, whether blood in the stool is caused by these sorts of problems.

Crohn's disease and ulcerative colitis are other relatively common causes of blood in the stool. And, as before, people with these illnesses tend to know about them. Patients with these long-term problems have abdominal bloating, often a mixture of diarrhea and constipation, and a combination of mucus and blood in the stool, while generally feeling unwell. These illnesses are intermittent, and flare-ups are often closely related to periods of high anxiety or stress.

The diagnostic tests for Crohn's disease and ulcerative colitis are similar to those used to detect bowel cancer. Usually, the doctor starts with a sigmoidoscopy, which involves looking directly into the lowest part of the large intestine. If Crohn's disease or ulcerative colitis is present, the lining of the colon will be sore, red, and inflamed. Sometimes doctors need to look further into the bowel; this is done with a colonoscopy. During this investigation, the whole length of the large intestine can be viewed, as far as the appendix (where the small intestine begins).

Exactly the same approach is often used if a doctor is trying to rule out colon cancer; in addition, the patient may be given a barium enema followed by X rays of the bowel, so that any growths can be detected. These tests will rule out or confirm the presence of cancer in the large intestine. To see whether there is a tumor in the small intestine, a different test (a barium swallow) and follow-through are required. They are based on exactly the same principle as the barium enema, but the radio-opaque material is swallowed rather than introduced into the body through the anus.

When a diagnosis of Crohn's disease, ulcerative colitis, or polyps has been made, the patient should undergo regular screening to watch for bowel cancer; it is more common in people with these conditions than in those with normal bowels.

Persistent diarrhea or unexplained constipation should also be checked, as these too can be symptoms of cancer. More commonly, though, they are found to be due to irritable bowel syndrome, spastic colon, or just poor diet.

Urinary Problems

Prostate cancer, where the enlarged gland presses on the urethra (the outflow tube from the bladder), can cause men to experience difficulty passing urine. This symptom is very common, especially in older men. Mostly it is caused by a benign growth of the prostate gland known as *benign prostatic hypertrophy*. Men who have difficulty passing urine are referred to a urologist, who will ascertain first if the prostate gland has grown, and second whether the growth is benign or malignant. A blood test to measure levels of prostatic specific antigen (PSA) can help to establish the presence of prostate cancer. The doctor will then usually perform a rectal ultrasound test, during which it is customary to take needle biopsies for analysis under the microscope.

As previously mentioned, it is better to avoid biopsies if possible, and if cancer can be diagnosed through the PSA and rectal ultrasound scan alone, this is preferable.

Difficulty passing urine in women should also be taken seriously, especially if it is painless. If there is pain, any bleeding is more likely to be caused by infection. But if not, there may well be a mass of some sort blocking the flow. In this case, the likely course of action would be a pelvic ultrasound.

Blood in the urine of both men and women should always be taken seriously. The most common cause is infection, but it can be caused by cancer in the kidney, ureter (tube from the kidney to the bladder), bladder, or urethra. If infection has been ruled out or treated and bleeding still persists, the bladder can be examined directly by undergoing a cystoscopy or bladderosocopy (visual examination of the bladder). The kidney, ureter, and bladder can also be looked at by ultrasound investigation, or by injecting into a vein in the arm a dye that can be seen on an X ray of the abdomen, revealing any problems throughout the urinary tract.

Weight Loss

If nothing else in your life has changed particularly, if you are eating and exercising as usual, and you suddenly lose a significant amount of weight with no obvious explanation, this ought to be investigated. You should start to be concerned if you lose between 7 and 14 pounds. Sudden weight loss can occur due to emotional traumas such as bereavement or the breakup of a relationship, or over excitement at the beginning of a new one. Stomach bugs can also cause quite marked weight loss, as can a change in diet. For example, people who change from a high-meat and high-fat diet to a vegan diet often lose a considerable amount of weight. Sudden weight loss may also occur if a new medication is started, such as a diuretic, which causes excess fluid to be passed out of the body in the urine.

If none of these situations apply, and weight loss has occurred for no obvious reason, it is best to get checked over by your doctor. He or she is likely to perform blood tests to look for cancers such as lymphoma and leukemia. A liver-function blood test will show if there is cancer affecting the liver. If severe weight loss occurs, it is possible that there is already secondary cancer in the body affecting the liver or lungs. But weight loss may occur with primary bowel cancer that is affecting the normal bowel habit or making eating and absorbing food difficult. It is therefore likely that the physician will do a physical examination of the abdomen or send a patient for an ultrasound check of the abdominal organs to rule out the presence of cancers of the pancreas, liver, kidneys, ovaries, or uterus.

Fatigue

Fatigue as a symptom is even more nonspecific and is linked to a whole range of health problems. In fact, Tired All The Time syndrome (TATT) is believed to be the most common problem currently presented in doctor's offices in the UK. In the general population, fatigue is usually the result of a combination of high stress, low exercise, and poor diet, often aggravated by toxins from smoking and drinking. The next most common cause of fatigue is postviral fatigue, which can occur after a nasty virus infection. In some cases, this goes on to become full-blown ME (myalgic encephalomyelitis), causing extreme exhaustion and muscle weakness.

When fatigue is associated with cancer, it may be a sign of quite advanced disease. But many people with cancer say that, looking back, they had been feeling excessively tired for six months or even a year before being diagnosed. Fatigue should always be taken as a serious warning that all is not well and that it is time to take active steps to recover a healthy balance in life. Ways of doing this will be addressed fully in Chapter 4. However, if your fatigue does not fit with any obvious pattern or explainable cause, then a doctor should assess you in the same way as for weight loss.

Difficulty Swallowing and Nausea

If you experience ongoing difficulty swallowing that cannot be put down to a sore throat or laryngitis, you should get the problem investigated without delay. Difficulty swallowing or regurgitating food is often associated with a growth in the esophagus, which must be treated as quickly as possible.

If eating often results in your feeling nauseous, or if food just won't digest and keeps repeating on you, it is possible that the outflow of food through the stomach or the small intestine is being impeded by a tumor. Once other causes of nausea—such as morning sickness, upset stomach, reaction to alcohol or drugs, and so on—have been eliminated, your physician is likely to refer you for an endoscopy to look directly at the gullet and stomach. If the result is negative, it will probably be followed by a barium swallow and follow-through and X rays to look at the state of the small intestine.

If the bowel becomes completely obstructed by a tumor, this will result in severe abdominal pain and vomiting, and should be treated as a medical emergency (see "Unexplained Abdominal Swelling," on the next page).

Headaches and Neurological Problems

Severe headaches are another nightmare area for physicians. The cause of a severe headache can range from a hangover or tension at one extreme, to meningitis or brain cancer at the other, both of which can be fatal. However, meningitis and brain cancer are both relatively rare in comparison with the number of headaches that occur due to tension, migraine, hangovers, nonserious viruses or bacterial infections anywhere in the body, or for no apparent reason at all. This means that a doctor has to be pretty worried before referring someone for a scan to look for a brain tumor. It is therefore quite important, if you have a strong suspicion that a headache is very odd, that you persist and convince your doctor that you really are worried.

A doctor will always act if there are accompanying neurological symptoms—signs indicating that the brain or other parts of the nervous system are malfunctioning in some way, such as when eyesight, hearing, balance, speech, smell, taste, muscle strength, or sensation in any part of the body become affected. There may also be unexplained fits, vomiting, mental changes, or even loss of consciousness. These symptoms will alert the physician that something could be causing pressure in the brain and must be investigated immediately.

Unexplained Abdominal Swelling

If the abdomen has swollen up in an uncharacteristic way, a doctor will want to check that there are no big masses causing this problem. Abdominal masses can be caused by tumors in the uterus, ovaries, bowel, liver, and, occasionally, the pancreas or kidney, or by lymphoma. Masses in the abdomen are not always cancerous; they can be caused by large fibroids in the uterus, for example, that are completely benign. The other cause of abdominal swelling that can be associated with cancer is ascites. This is when the abdomen fills up with fluid, caused by a diseased liver.

The abdomen can also swell for other noncancerous reasons, including gas accumulation, fluid retention, and, of course, pregnancy. A doctor should first examine the abdomen and perform a vaginal or rectal examination as well, if necessary. If diagnosis is still unclear, the patient is likely to be referred for abdominal ultrasound or an abdominal X ray. If any possibility of pregnancy exists, X ray should be avoided in favor of ultrasound.

Sometimes, if the gut has become obstructed or blocked altogether, abdominal swelling is an emergency problem. In this situation, a person will suffer severe colicky pains and quite often nausea or vomiting, and it is best to go straight to the emergency room or call an ambulance. Obstruction may be caused by severe constipation, at one extreme, or cancer, at the other; but must be treated quickly to avoid perforation of the bowel and peritonitis (infection of the abdominal cavity).

Vaginal Bleeding

At some time or other, premenopausal women will experience an occasional occurrence of irregular bleeding between periods. However, persistent intermittent spotting between periods must be checked by a doctor. In particular, any bleeding at all after menopause should be investigated right away. Doctors will check for cancers of the vulva, vagina, cervix, endometrium (uterine lining), uterus, or ovaries. Investigation may start with a vaginal examination, which may proceed to a colposcopy, during which the vagina is opened quite widely with a fixed speculum so that the cervix can be viewed directly by the naked eye or through a microscope. If any abnormalities are present, it may be necessary to take a sample of the uterine lining in a procedure known as a D and C (dilation and curettage). This may be backed up by ultrasound examination of the fallopian tubes and ovaries and/or a laparoscopy, where the pelvic organs are looked at directly through a keyhole incision in the abdominal wall.

SELF-EXAMINATION

Self-examination for the symptoms of cancer is really an extension of getting to know your body and taking good care of yourself in general. There are many areas of the body you cannot check yourself, but you can easily keep an eye on some parts.

It is a very good idea to check your skin regularly. If possible, get a partner, family member, or friend to check the areas that are difficult for you to see, perhaps while changing clothes at a gym or swimming pool.

Get used to the normal consistency of your breasts. This applies to both men and women; although rare, breast cancer can occur in men too. To do this, lie down flat on your back, raise overhead the arm on the same side as the breast you're checking, and with your other hand palpate the four quadrants of the breast separately, sensing whether there are any lumps or bumps beneath the surface. (Use the fingertips of a flattened hand for the most reliable sensing method.) Then feel the neck and underarm to check for any obvious lymph-gland swelling. Some masses or cysts in the breasts are normal; any changes should be investigated by a doctor. In addition, stand in front of a mirror and raise your arms overhead; then look at your breasts from all angles to check for any dimpling, pulling, or puckering of the skin. For women, it is best to examine the breasts during the few days immediately following the end of the menstrual period, when breast size and shape are least affected by the natural hormone cycle.

The groin should be checked the same way from time to time, for signs that could alert you to problems in the abdomen or legs.

For men, it is a good idea to check the testicles regularly. Grip the scrotum in such a way that you immobilize the testicles, and then feel each one all over its surface to make sure that all the contours are smooth and that you feel no lumps or bumps.

It is also a good idea to check your abdomen from time to time. Lie on your back with your knees bent and your feet flat on the floor or bed, then check the lower, middle, and upper abdomen to make sure there are no lumps or masses within the abdominal cavity. However, be aware that if you are very constipated, this can give the feeling that masses are present in the abdomen.

Another good idea, especially if you are a smoker and/or a drinker, is to look regularly within your mouth and at your lips to make sure no sores have formed that appear not to be healing.

SCREENING

Currently in the United States, most doctors perform routine screening for breast, cervical, and colorectal cancers, as well as manual exams for prostate and testicular cancer. In addition, doctors often will perform a PSA (prostate specific antigen) blood test on men over fifty to check for evidence of prostate abnormality. Otherwise, it is really a matter of being alert to symptoms that may appear or abnormalities that may be found during self-examination. Above all, it is absolutely vital to trust your "inner voice" or gut feeling if you sense something is really wrong, and to get yourself tested appropriately until you're either proved right or fully reassured.

Breast Cancer

An annual mammogram (X-ray examination of the breasts) is routine for all women in the United States who are over age thirty-five or forty and under the regular care of a physician. An annual manual examination of the breasts by a doctor or nurse is also recommended for women of all ages, as is monthly self-examination. Women at any age should go for a medical checkup immediately if they find any change in a breast.

Mammograms can identify breast tumors before they can be found by manual examination, but the procedure is controversial because of concern that repeated X rays of the breasts may contribute to cancer in those who do not have it. Many women prefer a combination of ultrasound screening and manual examination. But none of these three tests is foolproof; diagnosis has been missed with all three, and the risks of ultrasound are not yet fully understood. There is definitely a need for safer methods of breast cancer screening to be developed that are more accurate, with less potential hazard.

If you have a strong family history of breast cancer, or a genetic susceptibility, it is likely that you will be offered (or should ask for) mammography screening starting at a much younger age than your mid-thirties. If you are invited to have a mammogram, it is certainly advisable to take the opportunity, because cancers that are detected in this way, before they are even palpable as a lump, are usually curable. This is because, at this early stage, spread has not usually occurred further into the breast or into the neighboring lymph nodes, and there are no accompanying metastases. If early breast cancers can be removed completely, the chances of cure are very high.

Cervical Cancer

Another part of the body that is routinely screened is the cervix. Because cancer of the cervix affects both younger and older women, screening in the form of a Pap smear is done annually throughout a woman's life (if, that is, she makes regular visits to her doctor). Again, it is wise to have a Pap smear once a year, because the test can detect abnormalities in the cervix before they become cancerous. In this case, the lab report will indicate that there are either viral changes or CIN (cervical intraepithelial neoplasia) 1, 2, or 3; these changes should be taken seriously. Not everybody who has viral changes or CIN will definitely get cancer, but at least 10 to 20 percent of CIN 3 cervixes will become cancerous. If treated properly at this early stage, the condition will most likely not result in further problems.

Colorectal Cancer

Many U.S. doctors routinely screen their patients who are over age fifty for colorectal cancer with a test known as *flexible sigmoidoscopy* (*flex-sig* for short). There is a case for earlier screening if you have a familial history of adenomatous polyposis (polyps) or have one or more close relatives with colorectal cancer; if you have GI symptoms or rectal bleeding; if you have had a previous colorectal cancer that has been removed; if you have a history of ulcerative colitis, Crohn's disease, or breast, uterine, or ovarian cancer; or if you have had radiation treatment to the pelvis. Screening will involve rectal examination, testing for blood in the stool, sigmoidoscopy, colonoscopy, and possibly a barium enema.

Genetic, or "Family," Cancers

Most cancers are not hereditary. Even when more than one case of cancer appears in a family, it is more often than not just sheer coincidence. However, occasionally people do inherit an extra risk of developing the disease.

Inherited gene defects can cause a small proportion of breast and ovarian cancers, through the BRCA2 and, more rarely, BRCA1 genes. About 10 percent of bowel cancers are inherited, and a further 1 percent arise as a result of inherited familial adenomatous polyposis, which is initially a benign condition but can become malignant. Retinoblastoma—a form of childhood eye cancer—is inherited in four out of ten cases, and melanoma can also run in families. All these conditions can be screened for.

However, even if you have a family history of cancer, your risk may not be as high as you think it is. Individual risk depends a great deal on how old your relatives were when diagnosed and how closely related they are to you. The younger a person is when diagnosed, the more likely it is that the cancer is due to a genetic predisposition.

In order to assess your risk of developing cancer, it is necessary to compile a family tree, indicating all close relatives who have had a cancer. From this information, a calculation of your risk can be made and advice given on what screening might be appropriate.

If a certain form of cancer seems to run in your family, particularly if it tends to develop at a young age, you should talk it over with your doctor. You should discuss whether you need to be referred for additional testing in the hospital or at a clinic where people at potential risk are identified, counseled, and screened (see the Resources section at the back of the book for more helpful information).

4

❖

How to Revolutionize Your Physical Health

The first three chapters presented an in-depth look at cancer: how common it is, its causes, its risk factors, and medicine's relative ineffectiveness in treating it—all of which perhaps made pretty alarming reading. It is now time to look at the positive side of the story. There are many actions we can take in daily life that can help protect us against the development of cancer. Cancer prevention really comes down to understanding these factors and learning how to boost the body's ability to protect itself against cancer.

A famous comment by Louis Pasteur is relevant to cancer prevention. After a lifetime of studying bacteria and the course of infectious diseases he announced quite simply on his deathbed, "*Le terrain est tous,*" literally, the soil, or terrain, is everything. What he meant, perhaps, was something like this: "Yes, it is wonderful to have vaccinations to deal with infections, but it is actually a combination of the body's internal environment and our external environment that determines our susceptibility to infection. Only by working with the 'terrain' or environment can we hope to tackle infectious illness."

Pasteur turned out to be quite right. Over the years, the two things that have made the biggest difference in death rates from infectious diseases are the creation of proper sewage systems and a rise in the nutritional standards of the general public. Vaccinations alone were never going to be the answer to the problem of widespread infectious disease.

With cancer we have an identical situation. We will never eradicate cancer with medical treatment. Somehow, governments and research institutes all over the world seem to have missed this point. To date, billions of dollars and pounds have been poured into investigating cancer's causes and developing cancer treatment, while only a tiny fraction of the total research budget has been dedicated to cancer prevention and to helping to change our personal or collective environments. At the moment, developed countries spend more than 90 percent of cancer research budgets on cancer treatments and causes and only about 5 percent on prevention; the rest is spent on research into cancer care.

The point is that cancer, in most cases, is a preventable disease for which we know the main causes. But it will take a determined and concerted effort, and a much more responsible attitude by individuals and society as a whole, to tackle the problem head-on and to change the cancer picture.

It is time to get active and revolutionize your health and life by embarking on the holistic approach to cancer prevention. The first step in this process is to learn how to take control of the key factors that affect health and resistance to disease. These key factors are:

- ❖ healthy eating and cooking

- ❖ vitamin, mineral, and herbal supplements

- ❖ exercise

- ❖ dealing with stress, anxiety, and overwork

- ❖ sleep, rest, and relaxation

- ❖ maintaining high energy levels

- ❖ achieving peace of mind

To help you understand why these factors are so crucial to health, I will begin with a full explanation of the holistic model of health and illness. This will clarify why it is crucial to address health at all levels of body, mind, and spirit in order to prevent cancer.

THE HOLISTIC APPROACH TO HEALTH

The idea that our body's physical health is related to our states of mind, body, spirit, and environment has been around for centuries. However, with the advent of science and Newtonian physics, there was a distinct shift toward a model of medicine wherein the body was seen either as a machine with parts that could be fixed if broken, or as a collection of chemical mechanisms that could be controlled artificially with manmade chemicals. This approach, which reached its zenith in the late twentieth century, has been responsible for some astounding progress in medicine, bringing with it the possibilities of such things as hip replacements, cataract removal, organ transplants, and the controlling of many diseases through medication.

However, since the 1960s there has been great dissatisfaction with the idea of treating only the symptoms of disease without addressing the underlying causes. Strong interest has resurged in the idea that mind, body, and spirit are connected, and that each individual is connected to the whole of life and therefore to all other individuals. During the 1960s and 1970s, these "alternative" ideas were ridiculed and opposed by orthodox doctors. But during the 1980s and 1990s, hard scientific evidence emerged that has forced people to take seriously the holistic model of health and illness.

The key message of the holistic approach is that, far from being simply human machines made up of a complicated set of parts and chemicals, we are very complex beings, and the functions of our mind, body, and spirit really do interact, profoundly affecting our health and well-being. For example, nutrition affects not only our physical health but also our IQ and mental state. Exercise can radically change our mood, while meditation (which calms the mind) has a profound affect on the heart, breathing, and immune function. It has also been shown that spiritual healing changes the brain-wave pattern from stressed-out beta activity into self-healing alpha activity and raises the level of the immune "natural killer" cells that are so crucial in the body's fight against cancer. (See "Achieving and Maintaining High Energy Levels," on page 170, for a more thorough discussion of spiritual healing.)

But perhaps most extraordinary is the effect of prayer—which in scientific trials is shown to significantly improve the chances of survival after a heart attack—and the technique of visualization, which if used during chemotherapy can significantly extend the survival time of cancer patients. Visualization is a "mind over matter" technique whereby, in the "mind's eye," individuals literally picture themselves getting well or experiencing good outcomes from treatment. In addition, when people with cancer are helped to express their feelings of anger, grief, and disbelief in support groups, this too has been shown to have a positive affect on their survival. Early studies showed that people who demonstrated a positive "fighting spirit" when diagnosed with cancer survived up to 60 percent longer than those who collapsed and became "helpless and hopeless." More recently, studies of cancer patients consistently show that the prognosis is far worse for those who are depressed and helpless than for those who cope better mentally.

The Mind/Body Connection

Our understanding of the mind/body connection has greatly progressed during the last few years. From the 1950s to the 1970s we had only a very basic understanding of how stress and fear adversely affect body function. What was known was that stress or fear causes adrenaline to be secreted, which in turn prioritizes the functioning of the brain and muscles for the well-known "fight or flight" response: When we are frightened or stressed, activity in the body is diverted away from the "housekeeping" functions such as digestion, absorption, growth, immune response, healing, and repair. As a result, we are either mentally alert and physically strong, able to fight off the current threat or danger—or to run like hell!

This short-term stress response is highly advantageous to our survival. If a tiger chases you, digesting your breakfast or warding off infection is not exactly your or your body's highest priority! But if stress becomes prolonged or chronic, it can have a disastrous effect on health, because your system's vital "housekeeping" functions become compromised in the long term. Many of us live our lives in pronounced states of anxiety or fear, as if we were constantly being chased by a tiger—whether it be in the form of a bank manager, taxman, mortgage company, or our boss!

During periods of prolonged stress, the body maintains high cortisol levels and high adrenaline levels. Cortisol, the natural steroid secreted by the adrenal glands, helps us deal with challenging situations, but high cortisol and adrenaline levels also directly inhibit our immunity to disease and infection. This has been clearly demonstrated both in the laboratory and in real life. Stress has an adverse effect on blood pressure, cholesterol, and fat levels in the blood, and is associated with irritability and an increased dependence on cigarettes, alcohol, and drugs, with all their attendant problems.

Our increased understanding of the stress factor during the 1960s and 1970s explained why prolonged stress and high levels of fear are so deleterious to the body, but it did not explain why emotions affect our health so strongly. People started to ask, "Why does falling in love cause eczema or irritable bowel syndrome to clear up?" and "How can an old person die within weeks of his or her spouse dying, when there is nothing apparently wrong with him or her?" Nor did it explain why visualization and other mind-over-matter techniques have such a profound effect on our physiology.

The real revolution in our understanding of the mind/body connection is in the new scientific field of psychoneuroimmunology (PNI). This revolution started in the 1970s with Dr. Candace Pert's discovery of a receptor in the brain for a substance resembling morphine. Shortly after this, the substance itself was discovered and named *endorphin* or *enkephalin*. The discovery of this naturally occurring opiate in the brain triggered the discovery of more than two hundred other tiny messenger chemicals, substances named *neuropeptides* or *informational substances*. It was quickly realized that these substances are secreted not only in the brain and nerve tissue but also in all the other parts of the body.

From these revolutionary developments, it became clear that the old model of a brain and nervous system communicating only through neurotransmitters at the ends of the nerves was completely out of date. It was replaced by a model in which all the tissues of the body are able to communicate with each other through informational substances. This new approach is based on the knowledge that receptors for the messenger chemicals were found simultaneously in the brain and many other tissues of the body. The pathways of the neuropeptides were tracked, which revealed that there is a communication loop from the brain to the tissues and back again. Amazingly, the tissues "talk" to the brain just as much as the brain "talks" to the tissues! But more than this, it is now clear that the body's tissues can also communicate with each other.

These concepts are so revolutionary that they have completely blown apart the idea of the body as five separate anatomical systems working more or less independently (as was taught in medical schools for the last century). In fact, communication between all the systems of the body is so complex that even trying to imagine it is difficult. Bearing in mind that computers work on a binary system of two digits, that the whole of Western music is composed on a scale of twelve intervals, and that the English language is based on twenty-six letters, a neuropeptide communication system with a minimum of two hundred units provides more possible combinations than we can even begin to imagine.

In practice, different emotional states create certain patterns of neuropeptide secretion, which strongly affect tissue functioning within the body. When people are stressed, depressed, distressed, or emotionally repressed for long periods, the body's most common response is severe depression of immune function as well. This affects both the activity of individual immune cells and the number of circulating immune cells.

However, it is not just the immune system that is affected. Studies show that the red blood cells of people who are depressed and stressed carry less oxygen, and that a whole range of tissue functions changes according to one's predominant state of mind. Scientists have not yet worked out exactly how the mind-over-matter techniques of visualization and affirmation affect tissue functions, but circulating blood-cell levels have been shown to change in response to a person's visualization of an increase in their number. Thus it is clear that these techniques have very real physical consequences.

So where does this all fit into the prevention of cancer? Studies to date that look at whether there is a link between cancer and stress and distressing life events, have had conflicting results: Some show definite links, others do not. What PNI scientists now tell us is that it is not stress or distress per se that is the problem; it is how an individual reacts to it. A concept known as "personality hardiness" is used to describe people who respond positively to stress and difficult situations, seeing them as an exciting challenge and a source of potential empowerment, rather than succumbing to anxiety, fear, and feelings of powerlessness.

Certainly, people who are depressed, isolated, and socially dis-advantaged have higher rates of cancer and die more quickly from cancer than those who are happy, affluent, and well supported. This fits with the observation that people who become helpless and hopeless when they are diagnosed with cancer fare much worse than those with fighting spirit. From this evidence—and from studies that show that cancer patients who express their feelings in support groups live longer, and that visualization can extend survival time—it is clear that state of mind has a great deal to do with the body's ability to defend itself against cancer.

This is not the same as saying that psychological factors cause cancer or that people are in any way to blame if they get cancer. The bottom line is that the Western lifestyle is extremely stressful, and those who are prone to feeling anxious, helpless, and hopeless or who have lost their way in life are likely to be both more vulner-able to serious illness and at greater risk if they get one. What is important to note is that these ways of reacting to life can be changed—through a combination of psychotherapy, support, and self-help. How to go about doing this will be addressed fully in the next two chapters.

To be really well, the body's physical needs must also be met, by eating healthy food and taking food supplements, by enhancing our energy and vitality, by expressing our sexuality, and by getting enough exercise, rest, and relaxation. Fulfilling these needs enables us to free our bodies from the effects of fear and stress. Most of all, we must achieve peace of mind, making sure we have the most lively immune system possible. To do this, the primary aspect we must address is our state of mind and spirit.

Achieving Peace of Mind

The study and practice of meditation is a direct approach to achieving peace of mind. Meditation really is the most effective of the self-help techniques. In addition to producing profound benefits for immune function, it calms and strengthens the cardiovascular, nervous, gastrointestinal, and respiratory systems. Certainly, meditating will calm the emotions and lift a person's mood and spirit, and will lead to clearer thinking and far more efficient and effective work. Another way to achieve peace of mind is to deal directly with the stress of our busy lives. Both approaches will be addressed in full later in this chapter. Sometimes, however, peace of mind cannot be achieved until the state of our spirit is tackled head-on.

Freeing the Spirit

If you have become dispirited, or your spirit has been crushed or broken by life due to a combination of disappointment, grief, and frustration, or perhaps simply because you have not found a way to fully express yourself, this can have a very depressing or even devastating effect on the immune system. This explains why an elderly person may die within six weeks of losing his or her spouse; for when the will to live has gone, the physical body may very quickly give up as well.

Sadly, many people nowadays exist in an unfulfilled state, with very little sense of purpose or meaning in their lives and no real source of spiritual nourishment or emotional well-being. Often people live their lives based on the expectations and demands of others, having very little excitement or passion to enliven and vitalize them. Certainly, in the field of holistic cancer medicine, it is clear that when people lose the will to live or have no exciting, creative focus for their energy, no medicine, orthodox or complementary, will make them well. On the other hand, if a sense of purpose and passion is rekindled, their immune system is also revitalized and they rapidly get well from the inside out.

To free the spirit, it is often necessary to work on several fronts simultaneously. To start with, it is important to attend to our "emotional hygiene." Many of us tend to repress our feelings, holding on to anger, hurt, guilt, grief, and disappointment. These emotions then sit in the body, affecting our posture, breathing, and tissue functioning through PNI mechanisms, and weighing down and burdening our spirit.

Once you start to tune into these things, it is very easy to see the emotions that other people are hanging on to. If you look closely, you will see that their body language, breathing pattern, eyes, and facial expressions say it all! In holistic medicine, there is a saying, "What the mind represses the body expresses." We literally "embody" the feelings we can't let go of. Shedding old emotions and, more importantly, learning how to express rather than repress them, are crucial steps on the path to good health.

The next step is identifying what drives our behavior. Often, we are programmed from childhood to push ourselves relentlessly in order to achieve success, win approval, love, and affection, or achieve the perfection we think is expected of us or that we expect of ourselves. Much of the time we behave the way we think other people want us to, and our own unique spirit becomes submerged. Often this is linked to low self-esteem and a tendency to take care of others while neglecting or abandoning ourselves. Once we identify the slave driver, perfectionist, workaholic, or approval-seeking sides of ourself, the next task is to replace this programming with kinder, more encouraging, and supportive messages that allow our real selves to emerge and flourish and our spirits to lift.

This brings us to another fundamental feature of the holistic approach to health—the belief that healthy living and spiritual development revolve around having a healthy relationship with yourself, with others, and with the environment in which you live. It is staggering how many people put themselves at the very bottom of their list of people to care for. Sometimes they're not on the list at all. Many people look after their houses, cars, and pets far better than they look after themselves! Getting the relationship with yourself right will provide a solid foundation for everything else. If you take time to listen and respond to your own needs, and gradually work toward being true to yourself, your life and health will be transformed beyond recognition.

To take this process further, spend time in retreat, counseling, psychotherapy or supportive group work, or simply quiet down and listen to your inner voice: Discover what your core values and needs really are. It is vitally important to be involved in things that express your true self, because those things are what give you a sense of purpose, meaning, and value. Over time, try to work toward living in the right place in the right way, with a lifestyle, home, and job that truly reflect who you are.

It is also important to ensure that you can both express love and receive the love you need. You can do this in a number of ways: through personal relationships, through meaningful links with community or spiritual groups, through a strong belief in the work you do. By redefining your core values and priorities on a regular basis, you will be able to organize your life so that it reflects these values, and you give attention, priority, energy, and time to the really important things in life rather than the trivial.

Closely linked to those endeavors is the fulfillment of personal spiritual needs: We must ensure that we receive the nourishment and uplift we need. It is important to get our hearts and minds out of the hurly-burly of everyday life and into communion with our spiritual nature and into connection with all that is around us. People suffer, often without even realizing it, from a deep spiritual malaise and a longing to touch the world of Spirit and "the kingdom of heaven within."

For many of us, everyday hassles can be transcended by going to places of great natural beauty or by getting in contact with nature. For others, exquisite music or the spontaneous excitement, joy, and beauty of small children can lift them out of their normal, preoccupied state of mind. Some tap into the essence of divine love through human love and committed relationships, or through service to others. Creativity and self-expression are also major sources of joy and spiritual well-being. And for yet others, spiritual connection and uplift comes through meditation or religious practice. Some have a more immediate or gnostic sense of spirituality, enabling them to feel quite palpably the presence and love of a Holy Spirit or Higher Power; others have their relationship with Spirit through religious belief and the faith this generates.

Many who attend the Bristol Cancer Help Centre say that the recognition of their spiritual nature and the defining and prioritizing of their spiritual needs are responsible for their healing. The profound transformation they undergo as a result of opening up to the spiritual dimension and developing a personal spirituality results in a wonderful new relationship to life and death, and in many cases results in a remarkable physical recovery as well.

If you are prepared to prioritize peace of mind and spiritual well-being, your life will become both simpler and enriched at the same time. You may feel you have "come home" in a profound and meaningful way. Most people who go through this process say they feel more and more alive and happier than ever before. Not only does their health improve greatly, but they also feel younger. This slowing down of the aging process is very noticeable in people who are fulfilled spiritually—a very real phenomenon that can be attributed to the effects of a positive state of mind, which creates measurable improvements in our immune system and tissue function.

The Energy Model of Health

Looking at the body's underlying energy and vitality is an important way to evaluate our state of health. In all traditional Eastern medicines, such as acupuncture, shiatsu, yoga, and tai chi, the aim is to work with this underlying energy or "life force," ensuring that all the different energies of the body are in balance and that the overall energy levels are high. In acupuncture and tai chi the energy is called *chi*, in shiatsu *ki*, and in yoga *prana*. The Western equivalent of this energy is found in homeopathy, where it is referred to as the "vital force."

It is actually quite easy, even without training in Eastern medicine, to sense whether a person's energy is basically in good shape. All of us make an "energy diagnosis" when we look at our houseplants, judging whether they are full of life and vitality or not. People with good *chi* radiate health and are a pleasure to be around, whereas those who are low in energy or whose energy is out of balance often feel draining or uncomfortable to be with.

Nowadays, with high-tech photographic techniques such as Kirlian photography (or the movie version of this which was developed in the UK by Harry Oldfield), it is possible to see the body's energy field and to visualize the subtle energy systems on which Eastern medicine is based. With new bioenergy measuring and treatment devices, such as the Russian Scenar or Kosmed device (see the Resources section), the body's energy levels can be measured and treated at the same time.

Through modern physics, we now know categorically that all matter is fundamentally made of energy, and that living systems produce electrical fields. Our Eastern ancestors knew this thousands of years ago; they used this knowledge to detect, assess, and rebalance the subtle energies of the body. In the West, owing to a combination of poor diet, alcohol, cigarettes, stress, overwork, overstimulation, and sedentary lifestyle, most of us only experience about half our potential energy.

It is often helpful to visualize our energy, imagining that we have a spectrum of energy levels from 0 percent to 100 percent (see the diagram on page 134). People are usually born with very high energy levels, as all parents of small children can testify! Over time, our lifestyles rob us of that vitality, leaving most of us only halfway up the energy scale. At that level, people become susceptible to minor illnesses such as colds, flu, and upset stomach, and, though generally able to work, they suffer from a lack of energy.

The Energy Model of Health and Illness

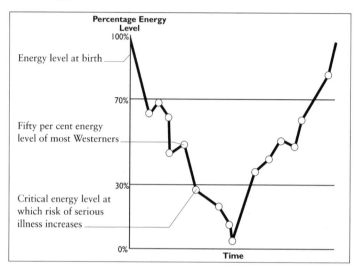

Overwork or adverse life events that cause upset, shock, or disappointment can make our energy levels dangerously low, to a critical level of, say, 30 percent. Below this point people are vulnerable to far more serious illnesses, and are likely to develop any health problem to which they are susceptible, whether it is asthma, schizophrenia, or cancer. Another problem is that when our energy level drops, our mental state changes also. When energy levels are low, self-esteem, confidence, and motivation go out the window. People are likely to become more fearful and anxious, to feel pain more acutely, to find it harder to sleep, and to feel that life is out of their control. In this situation they are on a slippery slope; they find it hard to pull themselves out of the trough they have fallen into. Indeed, at this point people often make things worse for themselves. When we feel things are getting out of control, our response is often to try harder, thereby stressing and exhausting ourselves even more. As a result, people become even more depleted and, at the same time, beat themselves up about their failure to "deliver."

A telltale sign of this low-energy state is that, even when we know what we need to do to increase our energy level, we are unable to do it. Many people who lead busy lives are in this state—they feel tired, exhausted, and demoralized. They know they would feel much better if they exercised, relaxed, or meditated but find it impossible to get to the gym or a meditation group. People in chronically low-energy states like this are vulnerable physically and psychologically, and are far more susceptible to developing cancer.

To reduce the risk of cancer in accordance with the energy model of health, we must learn how to "tune into" and assess our energy level, listen closely to what our body is telling us are the first steps we must take, and then adjust our behavior accordingly. The first and most obvious thing to do is to balance work with rest and recreation. It is also important to learn how to raise our energy level, through both therapeutic intervention and self-help techniques, which will be described later in this chapter.

As soon as our energy level rises, reaching, say, 70 percent, our psychological health starts to improve dramatically. People feel empowered—as if everything is going their way—and they often start to experience synchronicity or significant coincidences in their life. In other words, as the lift in energy raises their consciousness, they experience meaningful insight into their own lives and have a far greater sense of connection to and support from life itself. People repeatedly say that once in this state, life and the things they want *come toward them:* They no longer have to struggle constantly to make things happen.

When energy levels drop below the 30 percent level, it is usually necessary to receive therapeutic help to rebound. Therapies that can lift energy levels include acupuncture, shiatsu, homeopathy, and, especially, spiritual healing. Once energy levels are lifted out of the doldrums, it is possible to keep building them up through self-help techniques such as relaxation, meditation, tai chi, yoga, and exercise (see also the diagram on page 136). All these therapies and self-help techniques are described in more detail later in this chapter.

Recovering Vital Energy

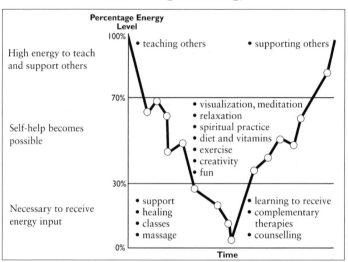

Caring for the Body

Combined with the spiritual, the other major factor within the holistic health model is taking care of ourselves physically. Eating properly and exercising regularly greatly affect our energy, vitality, and state of mind. But it is not just a matter of what food we eat, but also of where we shop, how we store food, how we cook food, and how we eat. We need to make changes to our diet that are sustainable, rather than alternating between periods of healthy eating and unhealthy binges.

Combining forms of exercise that build stamina with those that increase suppleness, strength, and harmonization of body, mind, and spirit is a good idea. The ideal combination is to get some form of aerobic exercise, preferably outdoors, once or twice a week, and to do a weekly class in yoga, tai chi, or chi gong as well, with a short daily practice of these disciplines at home.

CREATING YOUR OWN CANCER-PREVENTION PLAN

While reading the rest of this chapter you might consider making notes so that you can form your own cancer-prevention plan. As you read each section, try to make a list of the changes you wish to adopt and the methods you will use to achieve them.

Healthy Eating and Cooking

A whole-food organic diet, which emphasizes foods in their natural, unprocessed form and is very low in animal foods, fat, salt, sugar, chemical additives, stimulants (such as tea and coffee), and alcohol, is what we all should aim toward. For most people, this will mean dramatically increasing their intake of vegetables, fruit, grains, and legumes while reducing their total calorie intake, and changing everything "white" in their diet to the "brown" unprocessed equivalent. It will also mean drinking herbal teas, juices, and mineral or filtered water, rather than nonherbal tea or coffee.

Lynda McGilvray changed her diet completely after she was diagnosed with breast cancer at the age of thirty. Before the diagnosis in 1981, she never really thought about what she ate and often relied on fast food, leftovers, and ready-made meals. But after undergoing surgery and radiation, she attended the Bristol Cancer Help Centre in an attempt to find the support she needed. She was amazed at what she found there—everything made sense; it was a move that empowered her.

As well as learning meditation, relaxation, and healing, Lynda adopted a vegan diet suggested by the Centre. In the first six weeks after leaving the Centre, she made dramatic changes to her diet, cutting out all meat, fish, and dairy products and eating only vegetables and legumes. She also started taking a regimen of vitamins and mineral supplements. At first, these changes proved challenging for Lynda, whose children were young at the time. She felt like as soon as she had finished chopping vegetables for one meal, it was time to start on the next. But she persevered, and within two to three weeks felt cleansed, full of energy, and in control. After six weeks, she went back to eating fish and chicken occasionally, and now eats fish twice a week. Over the last eighteen years, Lynda's diet has changed, but she remains very aware of what she should and should not eat. Although days occur when she eats less well, these are far outnumbered by the good days.

Since the first diagnosis, Lynda has had two recurrences of breast cancer—in 1988 and 1996. But for the last four years there has been no sign of the disease, and at age forty-nine she feels very good. Being diagnosed with cancer—followed by the help she received from the Bristol Cancer Help Centre and her local cancer-support group—has completely changed Lynda's life. Now she enjoys a much better outlook and feels she has gained a great deal of her new vitality and continued good health from healthy eating.

How to Change the Way You Eat

Changing something as fundamental as the food you eat involves a great deal of commitment and support. It is important to make changes in a way that is sustainable. Quite often, if changes are too radical or too quick, they are abandoned within weeks, especially if the new regimen feels like a diet or a form of deprivation, leaving you with the desire to binge on "naughty" foods. The other ingredients for success include getting the right sort of support to help you make the changes, and acquiring the right information, recipes, and new cooking skills.

Support. If you are going to start eating in a healthy way, it is vital to enlist the support of your partner, family, colleagues, and friends. Also, if you are serious about making this commitment to yourself, it is good to have "witnesses." The very process of telling people will make your intention seem more real. Obviously, it is better still if you can get the people you live with to make the changes too. Doing so will prevent all sorts of conflicts about how you are going to shop, cook, and prepare food—and the more nitty-gritty issue of how the household budget is going to be spent! If you can't persuade your nearest and dearest to join in, you might enlist the aid of a "buddy" or even a small group of friends or colleagues who would like to make the changes with you.

If you can muster several people who also want to change their diet, you could form your own healthy-eating support group and meet regularly for a few weeks to talk about how you are doing and to swap information and creative ideas. I have seen this work in an office environment, where a whole team decided to clean up their act with regard to food. They supported each other by replacing cookies and cakes with big bowls of fruit, sugary drinks with mineral water and fruit juice, and tea and coffee with herbal teas. They also met weekly to discuss meal plans and their progress.

The group started with a spring-cleaning "detox" diet to lose weight that revolved around eating only fruit, steamed vegetables, salads, soup, and brown rice for six weeks. Thereafter, other whole foods were added. The group members were delighted with the results, both in terms of weight loss and a marked improvement in their energy levels and mental clarity. The feeling of solidarity among members was wonderful, and it rubbed off on their work together.

If you recognize that you have a great emotional dependency on food, you may find it necessary to get more than family or friends to support you; in such a case, going to a counselor or doctor may be a good idea. Once you start to eat fewer heavy foods, which are sedating, you may well uncover anxieties and feelings that have been lurking under the surface for years. If this occurs, it is unlikely that you will be able to change your eating patterns successfully until you get therapeutic help. Counseling can help people to offload their emotions and make long-term changes in the way they deal with their feelings. (Agencies through which you can find a counselor are listed in the Resources section at the back of the book.)

Information. Getting information about how to cook healthy food has never been easier. Healthy eating is talked and written about frequently these days, and many good cookbooks and nutrition books are available that offer step-by-step advice on what to do (see the Resources section). Before you start your new diet you will need the following:

❖ dietary advice explaining what to eat and what not to eat

❖ a clear idea of what healthy foods are available and what you should buy

❖ a meal plan to take you through the first few weeks

❖ nutritional information to ensure that you eat a balanced and healthy diet

❖ a good set of recipes

❖ professional advice if you have special dietary needs as a result of illness or disabilities

❖ information on how to store and cook foods to gain maximum nutritional value

This information will be detailed in the following pages. But if this all seems too much, the whole operation can be made far simpler by going to a nutritional therapist for one-to-one help in successfully changing your diet. A nutritional therapist is not the same as a dietician. Most dieticians are trained in the standard Western diet and how to adjust it for certain illnesses or conditions. They may happily recommend a diet based on meat, dairy foods, and refined carbohydrates. Nutritional therapists, by contrast, look at the role of food itself—as a cause and treatment of illness—and tend to advocate a whole-food, healthy diet. On the other hand, many registered dieticians *do* promote holistic and complementary therapies and *do* counsel people on good, preventive nutritional practices. Planning changes to your diet with a professional can make all the difference in your chances of success and is highly recommended. (See the Resources section for information on finding a nutritional therapist.)

Dietary Guidelines

Key advice for a healthy diet:

❖ Eat fruits and/or vegetables at every single meal. Include a high proportion of raw fruits and vegetables in your diet every day, either on their own, in salads, or as homemade juices, which are an excellent source of nutrition. (Most commercially available fruit and vegetable juices are pasteurized. Part of the pasteurization process involves heating the juice, which destroys health-giving enzymes, so the homemade variety is much better.) For making juices at home you will need a basic centrifugal juice extractor (costing around $75.00), or a better, more expensive juice press.

❖ Get as much variety in your diet as possible, and try different legumes, fruits, and vegetables. This will ensure that you get the full spectrum of minerals and vitamins and the vital plant phytochemicals necessary to prevent cancer.

❖ Replace refined and processed foods with the whole-food, unprocessed equivalent. This means replacing white bread with brown bread, preferably made from 100 percent whole-grain flour (check the ingredient label: If the first ingredient listed is enriched flour rather than whole-grain flour, that means there's more white flour in the bread than whole-grain flour, and you should select another brand); white rice with brown rice; white pasta with brown pasta; ordinary crackers with whole-grain varieties; sugary cakes and desserts with whole-grain, low-sugar versions; normal breakfast cereal with granola or whole-grain hot cereal; sweets and chocolate with nuts, dried fruits, or ordinary fruit; and sweetened drinks with mineral water or fruit or vegetable juice (preferably homemade).

❖ Replace red meat and farmed chicken and fish with vegetable protein from beans (including soy products), lentils, peas, quinoa, and other legumes; include occasional servings of deep-sea fish, wild salmon or trout, free-range organic chicken or game, free-range organic eggs—and the very occasional serving of organic red meat.

❖ Replace most animal fats with vegetarian equivalents. The exception to this rule are the fish oils, which contain essential omega-3 fatty acids. They are found in oily fish such as mackerel, herring, or salmon (wild), or you can take fish-oil tablets. Replace whole milk with organic skim milk or, better still, with vegetable drinks such as soy, oat, or rice milk.

You could try cutting milk from the diet altogether by drinking weak black tea and using fruit juice on granola for breakfast. Hot cereal can be eaten without milk, flavored with fruit concentrates or with maple syrup.

❖ Replace cheeses with vegetable dips and spreads, such as hummus (made from chickpeas/garbanzo beans), guacamole, and any of the many varieties of salsas now available. It is also better to use a fish pâté than cheese. Make sure dips are not full of hidden cheese or sour cream.

❖ Replace animal fat in cooking with vegetable oils—preferably organic cold-pressed olive oil or canola oil. Use specialty oils such as sesame oil and walnut oil for flavoring salad dressings.

❖ Replace cream with soy cream and ice cream with soy ice cream.

❖ Replace normal yogurts with soy desserts and yogurts, such as Tofutti.

❖ Replace butter with vegetable equivalents such as an olive oil-based spread. Many margarines are unhealthy because they are highly processed and contain hydrogenated and trans-fatty acids, produced by excessive heating of the fats during the production process. Brands of margarine that do not contain hydrogenated fatty acids include Spectrum and Earth Balance.

Faced with the above advice, most people panic that they will fail to get sufficient protein and calcium for healthy growth and bones. I like to remind people that huge creatures such as elephants and cows are vegetarian and have no problem maintaining their massive bone structure and good health.

In reality, most people in developed countries eat far too much protein every day. It is estimated that we actually need only 40 grams (just over 1 ounce) of protein per day to replace the wear and tear on our joints and muscles. All the basic vitamins and minerals we need are available from a varied vegan diet. Over the years, the meat and milk marketing boards have done a very good job of convincing us that good health depends on our intake of dairy foods, meat, and eggs. Just try to hold clearly in your mind the fact that most degenerative health problems in the West are due to overeating and, in particular, to the excessive consumption of animal fats and meat.

Buying Healthy Food

If the idea of eating whole foods is new to you, pay a visit to a good natural-foods grocery and see exactly what is on offer. You will be amazed by the huge selection of raw ingredients on display, as well as the ready-made vegan and vegetarian meals. Of course, many of these healthy foods, such as legumes, seeds, nuts, dried fruits, and whole-grain cereals, are available in supermarkets too. But since most supermarkets stock a much higher ratio of processed foods to whole foods, it is worth going to a specialty natural-foods market to familiarize yourself with the full range of what is available. Supermarkets are now paying heed to the healthy-eating message, however, and more and more are offering organic produce and other foods, so once you know what you are looking for, it may well be possible to return to your normal supermarket.

Cookbooks

Natural-foods markets will often have a book section, where you can pick from a full range of North and South American, European, and Asian vegetarian cookbooks. Quite often, Indian or Middle Eastern vegetarian cooking is a good option for those who are used to an elaborate diet and tend to think of vegetarian food as boring. The main problem with basic vegetarian meals is that they can at first seem bland in comparison with the intensity of flavors and the variation of textures involved in traditional cooking. However, the exotic recipes and the diversity of Asian or Latin American cooking methods and ingredients overcome this problem very well. As well, any good bookshop will have a vegetarian section in the cookbook department. (See the Resources section for cookbook suggestions.)

Whole-Foods Shopping

On your first trip to the natural-foods grocery or a good supermarket, a basic shopping list would include:

❖ brown rice, pasta, and flour

❖ dried beans, peas, and lentils

❖ sugar-free, high-quality granola and whole-grain hot cereal

❖ good-quality organic whole-grain bread

❖ nuts, seeds, and dried fruit

❖ vegetable spreads and dips, such as hummus

❖ herbal tea

❖ mineral water

❖ whole-grain crackers and desserts

❖ soy, oat, or rice milk

❖ soy yogurt or dessert

❖ olive-oil spread, or Spectrum or Earth Balance margarine

❖ extra-virgin olive oil

❖ tamari or soy sauce for flavoring foods (as an alternative to salt)

In addition to these basics, building up a selection of herbs, spices, and special ingredients is a good idea to help flavor vegetarian foods in interesting ways. Useful ingredients include garlic, ginger, balsamic vinegar and other flavored vinegars, chili powder, salsas, and sesame oil. It is also possible to buy soy mayonnaise, which is not nearly so high in saturated fat as ordinary mayonnaise. Excellent green and red curry pastes from Thailand are available, as are delightful flavorings such as lemongrass, star anise, and Chinese five spice, along with the fresh herbs cilantro, rosemary, thyme, bay leaves, and basil. Soy desserts mixed with fresh fruit can be made far more interesting by marinating the soy with vanilla pods and star anise, together with a little honey or maple syrup. Ripe tomatoes served with freshly chopped basil, olive oil, balsamic vinegar, and salt and pepper are an absolute delight.

Fruit concentrates, such as apple and strawberry, can be used very effectively to flavor sauces, desserts, and cakes, as can maple syrup. Soaking dried fruits with herbs is another delicious option. For example, soak Hunza apricots from Kashmir in India with bay leaves and cardamom seeds overnight, then bring them to a boil in just enough water to cover, and simmer for five to ten minutes. To thicken and enrich the juice, leave it to steep for a further twenty-four hours before serving. Served with soy-ice-cream, this dish is indeed proof that healthy food can be just as rich and delicious as more conventional food—and in no way equals deprivation!

An Introductory Meal Plan

The better the structure of a new diet, the more successful it is likely to be. A meal plan for one week is a good idea to begin with, and it can either be repeated or changed at the beginning of each new week.

Breakfast should include some of the following:

- ❖ fresh fruit, fresh fruit salad, or a dried fruit compote (soaked overnight)

- ❖ healthy cereal such as granola or hot cereal (which can be made from many other grains besides oats)

- ❖ brown toast with high-quality, low-sugar fruit spreads or honey

- ❖ boiled eggs (occasionally)

- ❖ fruit juice or herbal teas (if you are going to drink tea or coffee, try to do so only once or twice a day and drink herbal teas or mineral water the rest of the time; additionally, it is better for your teeth—and your children's teeth—to drink fruit juice at meal times only)

Decide which is going to be your main meal—lunch or dinner—and swap the following meals around accordingly. A light lunch could include a choice of:

❖ vegetable or fish soup

❖ green salad, bean salad, or rice salad

❖ a whole-food vegetarian pie, samosa, or falafel

❖ whole-grain bread or toast with hummus, tomatoes, and arugula (or other field greens)

❖ fresh fruit, fruit salad, or stewed fruit

For dinner you could choose from:

❖ whole-grain pasta with tomato or mushroom sauce, vegetarian bolognese sauce, or pesto

❖ vegetable curry or dal with brown rice

❖ stir-fried vegetables and tofu with brown rice

❖ vegetable stews, baked or stuffed vegetables

❖ whole-food fruit desserts, pies, pastries

All of the above should be accompanied by a fresh salad and/or steamed vegetables. It is also fine to include organic fish, poultry, or meat on an occasional basis.

Nutritional Information

A healthy diet includes a good balance of:

❖ protein

❖ carbohydrates (starch and sugar)

❖ essential fatty acids

❖ fruits and vegetables

Vegetarian protein comes from beans (including soy, which contains all twenty-one essential amino acids), peas, lentils, nuts, seeds, and the delicious cereal quinoa (which also contains all the essential amino acids). *Carbohydrates* are available from bread, pasta, rice, corn, potatoes, and other root vegetables. *Essential fatty acids* are obtained from nuts, seeds, vegetables, and fish oils. Within all these food groups, make sure you consume as much variety as possible. These healthy whole foods all contain a different balance of vitamins and minerals, and for optimum health it is best to vary your intake and experiment with new legumes, fruits, and vegetables. Jane Sen, of the Bristol Cancer Help Centre, says that an easy way to be sure you are getting the full range of nutrients is to mix vegetables and foods of different colors in one meal. If you are worried about getting the right nutritional balance, especially for children or the elderly, again the advice is to invest in some time with a nutritional therapist or buy a good book on whole-food nutrition (see the Resources section). The most important thing to remember is that you *can* get all the nutrients you need from a vegetarian diet.

Another concern people have about changing to a whole-food diet is that they will lose too much weight. It is usually true that when people make the change they initially lose some weight as they eliminate refined sugars and animal fats from their diet. For example, one candy bar can contain the same amount of sugar as about fifteen apples! However, people on a whole-food diet are satisfied long before eating this many apples, and therefore they consume far less sugar while getting all the healthy vitamins, minerals, phytochemicals, and fiber they need. After a while, weight normally reaches a healthy equilibrium. If it continues to fall, you are probably concentrating too much on fruits and vegetables and not getting enough carbohydrate and fat. In this case, it may be helpful to seek the advice of a nutritional therapist to find out where in your diet you can make adjustments.

A great added bonus of changing to a healthy cancer-prevention diet is that other illnesses you may have will start to clear up. The most common improvements are in asthma, eczema, arthritis, migraine, and stomach/intestinal complaints. Many of these illnesses are caused by allergies to animal foods, or by lack of the right minerals, vitamins, and plant phytochemicals—problems rectified by a healthy, vegetable-based diet. People also produce far less mucus, and the throat, ears, and sinuses feel much clearer. This means fewer infections. Other benefits include an increase in energy levels, clarity of mind, and healthy skin. In fact, most people who make these changes ask themselves why on earth it took them so long to do so, because they feel so much lighter and clearer, and so very much more alive.

Specific Anticancer Foods

All vegetables, nuts, seeds, and legumes contain some of the vital cancer-preventing phytochemicals, so eating the widest range possible of these foods is essential. However, some foods contain particularly high levels of these protective plant chemicals; you should make sure your cancer-prevention diet is high in these ingredients. This topic has been brilliantly researched by nutritionist Suzannah Olivier, who has compiled the following list of foods that help to prevent cancer. The full list of the phytochemicals they contain is in Appendix 5. For a full explanation of the scientifically researched properties of individual phytochemicals, I thoroughly recommend Suzannah Olivier's book *The Breast Cancer Prevention and Recovery Diet* (see the Resources section).

Anticancer foods: alfalfa; onions; spring onions; garlic; leeks; chives; almonds; apples; broccoli; cabbage; brussels sprouts; kale; bok choy; kohlrabi; arugula (rocket); horseradish; radishes; rutabaga; turnips; sprouted broccoli and cauliflower seeds; burdock root; citrus fruits; flaxseed oil; ginger; grapes; licorice; linseeds (flaxseeds); the Asian mushrooms maitake, reishei, and shiitake; nettles; almonds; walnuts; black walnuts; pecans; sunflower seeds; sesame seeds; olive oil; apricots; cantaloupe; carrots; yellow and red peppers; beets; squash; sweet potatoes; red and black berries; parsley; pineapple; potatoes; legumes and beans; brown rice; the seaweeds kombu, kelp, nori, arame, laver bread, dulse, and wakame; soy products; black tea; green tea; tomatoes; turmeric.

Learning New Culinary Skills

There is no way around the fact that changing to a whole-food, vegetarian diet will involve acquiring new skills. You may be fortunate enough to have access to a whole-food cooking class through a local college or cooking school. Local nutritional therapists may also teach or know about courses on whole-food cooking, as might the people who run local natural-foods markets, restaurants, or holistic-health clinics. Again, a good whole-food cookbook will offer many ideas and vital guidance on how to master these basic skills. But the simplest way is to find somebody who already eats healthily who can teach you the first steps. These will include learning to:

❖ cook brown rice, legumes, grains, and cereals successfully

❖ stir-fry and bake vegetables

❖ make a good variety of salads that include raw vegetables, seeds, nuts, fruits, and cooked legumes as well as the usual salad ingredients

❖ make vegetable soups and juices

❖ make whole-food cakes, cookies, and desserts.

❖ make basic sauces and dressings with healthy ingredients

Sustainability

In order to sustain the changes you make, the golden rule is to start adding healthy foods to your diet before you take other things out. For example, try first to get into the habit of eating fruits and vegetables with every single meal. The next step is to replace all processed "white" foods with their brown equivalents. Because these foods are so much more sustaining than their white counter-parts, you will soon start to find that your blood sugar is less inclined to dip, which is what makes you want to reach for sugary snacks and drinks. The desire to eat sugary or fatty snacks between meals will gradually reduce. Once this starts to happen, your appetite will level out and it will then be possible to eliminate or drastically reduce richer and heavier foods such as meats and ani-mal fats. In a short time you will feel so much better that you will wonder how you survived so long eating any other way.

Healthy Cooking

Barbecuing, smoking, and microwaving foods (especially meat and meat fats) are the cooking methods to avoid. It is also best to avoid overheating fat when frying and, in particular, to avoid the repeated use of oils for deep-frying. Overheated oils and smoke from barbecues and food-smoking processes produce dangerous free radicals in food, which can be carcinogenic. It is therefore advisable to keep clear of barbecued, smoked, and charbroiled meats and fish and to restrict frying to a minimum. When you do fry food, always use new oil and avoid heating it so long that it smokes. This is a sure sign that the fat is beginning to superheat and break down into free radicals.

The best cooking methods are:

❖ steaming

❖ stir-frying

❖ stewing

❖ roasting

❖ baking

With steaming and stir-frying, foods can be cooked quickly and lightly, thereby retaining much of their natural texture and nutrients. Baking, roasting, and stewing are gentler ways of cook-ing than frying or grilling and allow flavors to melt into one another at lower temperatures. Believe it or not, it is actually possible to "fry" foods in a little water. Heat a small amount of water in a frying pan and cook the food exactly as if you were frying it. You can then add good-quality cold-pressed oils (like olive, sesame, or walnut) at the end of cooking for flavor and nutritional value. By cooking this way, you will appreciate the flavor of the oil far more than when it is overheated and broken down in frying.

When stir-frying use a minimum amount of oil—just enough to keep vegetables or other foods from sticking to the wok or frying pan. Steaming is the healthiest cooking method because foods that are steamed retain maximum flavor and texture (in contrast to those that are boiled, which leak vital nutrients—particularly minerals—and flavors into the cooking water). With steaming, there is only a slight leakage of nutrients into the steaming water. Whether steaming or boiling food, it is a good idea to use the leftover cooking water in other recipes, such as soups, stews, and sauces.

When you change to healthy eating, one of the best things to master is how to make really good and varied salads. In the old days, people were brought up with the idea that a salad comprised lettuce, tomato, and cucumber. But in reality the range of possibilities is enormous. What works particularly well is grated raw vegetables mixed with conventional salad foods, sprouted seeds, and cooked legumes. Grated carrots and beets, finely chopped zucchini or broccoli, mixed with sprouts or watercress, field greens (such as arugula), and tomatoes, for example, make many stunning salads. Precooked beans are another good ingredient. Red kidney beans with chopped tomatoes, parsley, a little chopped onion, and a good garlic dressing make a very nutritious and delicious meal.

Try also making salads with grains such as rice, quinoa, bulgur wheat, or couscous (which is often mistaken for a grain but actually is a form of pasta), and experiment with different dressings. Most of us get locked into using oil and vinegar, but wonderful dressings can be made with other ingredients. For example, try puréed, peeled fresh tomatoes and basil with a little lime, lemon, or vinegar, salt and pepper.

Another good skill to acquire is the ability to sprout seeds and legumes. This can be done in jam jars or other glass containers. Or you can buy a sprouting kit, available at most natural-foods groceries. The secret is to first soak the seeds or legumes in double their volume of water for the first day, drain and rinse them on the second day, then leave them damp in the jar to germinate. Rinse them again each day until the sprouts are ready to eat. The best seeds and beans to sprout are alfalfa, mung, aduki, and chickpeas (garbanzo beans).

Useful Equipment

To make whole-food cooking easier, it is worth investing in a good food processor, because you will be preparing more vegetables and salads. A food processor will chop and grate vegetables extremely quickly. Also, invest in a juice extractor or press so that you can use pure vegetable and fruit juices, both for drinking and to make delicious sauces and soups. It is also a good idea to obtain a vegetable steamer. The most useful one is the collapsible model that fits inside an ordinary saucepan. It is circular with petals that open like a flower, so it fits in different size pans, and it is available from all good cookware shops and some supermarkets. If you have a large family and are likely to be doing a lot of steaming, you could invest in a more elaborate, multilevel steamer in which you can cook three types of vegetables simultaneously. A hand mixer can also be invaluable for making vinaigrettes, soups, or vegetable purées in the pan they've been cooked in, and for chopping herbs for sauces. If you can, get an electric coffee grinder too, but use it solely for grinding nuts, seeds, and spices such as nutmeg. A mortar and pestle can serve this purpose equally well.

For stir-frying, invest in a wok, which is what the Chinese use for most of their cooking. It looks a bit like a frying pan but has a gently curved shape and a long wooden handle. It is designed this way to make it easier to keep tossing the contents of the wok gently during cooking, which ensures that everything in the pan gets cooked quickly and evenly without burning or overcooking. A good set of knives, sharpened regularly, is essential for peeling and chopping vegetables, and another handy tool is a small mandolin-style vegetable peeler (which does the job much quicker than a standard peeler).

Vitamin, Mineral, and Herbal Supplements

The main vitamins, minerals, and plant-food supplements that protect against cancer are:

- ❖ the antioxidant vitamins C, E, and beta-carotene (the safe form of vitamin A)

- ❖ the minerals zinc and selenium (involved in the enzymes that are used in antioxidant processes)

- ❖ naturally occurring antioxidants and plant phytochemicals (condensed and sold as plant-food supplements)

- ❖ vitamin D (protects the bowel against cancer)

- ❖ low-dose aspirin (has also been shown to protect against bowel cancer)

Some people say it is not necessary to take vitamin and mineral supplements to prevent cancer if you are eating a healthy diet. But I disagree, because most of us are exposed to high levels of stress and chemical toxicity in the environment. I believe it is a good idea to take basic vitamin and mineral supplements to boost the immune system and provide background antioxidant support to our tissues.

Important: smokers should not take beta-carotene. Recent research has shown that while people with high blood levels of beta-carotene are protected against cancer, smokers who rapidly increase their levels of beta-carotene are more likely to develop lung cancer. The reason for this is not yet understood. My message to smokers is this: first, give up smoking (take vitamins and minerals during this process, as suggested on page 91); then, after around three months, add beta-carotene supplementation, when the smoke is well and truly out of your system.

Recent controversy in the UK about how consuming more than 500 mg of vitamin C per day can cause oxidative damage to

DNA has been misleading. Overall, there is still overwhelming evidence in favor of the use of vitamin C to prevent cancer. The suggestion that vitamin C can actually cause DNA damage is not supported by the scientists who did the trials themselves! These scientists say that oxidative changes seen in DNA with vitamin C, which could be construed as DNA damage, is the first of two steps in an overall DNA-repair process triggered by vitamin C.

Suggested supplements and dosages for cancer prevention and optimum health are as follows (IU = international units):

- ❖ vitamin C (500 mg three times per day)

- ❖ beta-carotene (15 mg per day), but not recommended for smokers

- ❖ vitamin E (400 IU per day). If you are taking anticoagulant drugs, let your doctor know you also plan to take vitamin E because it has a slightly anticoagulant effect

- ❖ selenium (200 IU per day)

- ❖ vitamin B complex (50 mg once per day)

- ❖ multivitamin/mineral tablets (one per day), which contain some vitamin D and zinc as well as the full spectrum of other minerals and vitamins needed to maintain health

By consuming at least one glass of freshly prepared vegetable juice every day, you will ensure that these supplements are used optimally by the body. All the naturally occurring cofactors and enzymes from the vegetables support the body's use of extra vitamins and minerals.

In good natural-foods markets, you will find products that have been designed with cancer prevention in mind. These contain a wide range of the phytochemicals, vitamins, and minerals that are known to be helpful, usually in the form of either powders or liquids to be taken daily. There is no doubt that these products will make you feel fantastic, as well as convey excellent protection. Of particular value are plant supplements that contain catechins, the elements of green tea that are so protective. Also available now, in tablet form, is the active anticancer ingredient from the brassica family. It is called *indole-3-carbinol*, and the daily protective dose is 300 mg. Two other food concentrates that significantly boost immune function and protect against cancer are MGN 3 (a mushroom extract) and IP6 (a derivative of vitamin B). Among other effects, they both significantly raise levels of the all-important immune "natural killer" cells, which are known to destroy cancer cells.

If your family history puts you at greater risk of bowel cancer, it is wise to take a vitamin D supplement and 300 mg of enteric-coated aspirin daily. This type of aspirin is designed to be broken down once it has gone through the stomach, helping to prevent stomach ulcers. Taking extra calcium and folic acid is also believed to reduce colon-cancer risk. Studies have shown that legumes and beans protect against uterine cancer and, astonishingly, that strawberries and raspberries protect against cancer of the cervix!

Protection against cancer of the prostate is achieved by taking vitamin E. Some scientists recommend 50 mg per day, which is around 75 IU. Others recommend as much as 800 IU. I recommend a level of 400 IU for both men and women as an important element of overall cancer prevention.

Anticancer herbs include essiac (an American Indian medicine that is widely available at healthfood stores and herbalists) and carctol (an Ayurvedic medicine, from India—see the Resources section for purchasing information). These can be taken at maintenance-dose levels as part of a cancer-prevention plan. Another intriguing proposition is to make and drink kombuchu, a sour drink believed to have anticancer properties. Like ginger ale, it is generated from a "plant" or culture that grows and requires dividing regularly.

Exercise

Exercise is a vital element of cancer prevention because it cleans out the tissues of the body. When we exercise, blood flow increases to all parts of the body, transporting oxygen, nutrients, and white blood cells to the tissues. This in turn promotes the flow of blood in both veins and lymph glands away from the tissues, taking toxins to the kidneys, liver, skin, and lungs for excretion. As previously mentioned, in traditional Eastern medicine, disease is believed to develop in areas of "stagnation" within the body. In acupuncture or shiatsu, this is seen as stagnation of energy, or *chi*. But the concept of stagnation can also be applied to a physical process—when, for example, tissues and joints literally clog up with toxins from our diet and from the breakdown products of alcohol, drugs, and cigarettes. Fat, calcium, heavy metals, and organic chemical residues from environmental pollution are deposited directly in the tissues, as are the breakdown products of radiation. So it is easy to see how tissues become more and more toxic, creating the ideal environment for cancer to develop. It is therefore not surprising that exercise lowers cancer rates. Statistically, women who exercise are 10 to 20 percent less likely to develop breast cancer than those who do not.

But which sort of exercise is best? In the holistic approach to health, Eastern exercises such as yoga, tai chi, and chi gong are favored. This is because they are intelligently designed to involve every single tissue, joint, and organ, bringing blood and vital energy to all parts of the body. In addition, they incorporate elements of relaxation, deep breathing, and meditation, which produce strong benefits through the mind/body connection. They can also generate a harmonious and respectful attitude to life, laying good foundations for the development of a spiritual practice.

Yoga is a multilevel process in which learning the postures (or *asanas*) is only one of the seven pathways toward complete health, happiness, "right living," and, ultimately, spiritual enlightenment. Of course, it is up to each individual how far he or she wishes to take the study of yoga. But even at the most basic level of attending a weekly class that combines a mixture of postures with some relaxation, meditation, and breathing exercises (*pranayama*), the benefits to health and well-being are phenomenal. One way to find an instructor is through the nonprofit Yoga Alliance; teachers and schools certified by the Yoga Alliance must meet minimum standards. The organization's website lists schools and instructors by state, province (in Canada), or country (see the Resources section).

Tai chi is the exercise you may have seen being practiced in a park by people in the early morning or in the evening. The benefits of tai chi go very deep, and its practice is highly recommended as a form of cancer prevention. Chi gong (also spelled *qigong* or *chi kung*) comes from the same roots as tai chi but tends to be used when people are already ill. *Chi gong* literally means "energy work," and the practice is usually tailored to the needs of individuals to help them rebalance and strengthen themselves in mind, body, and spirit in order to overcome a particular health problem. In the West, where many of us have allowed our physical health to degenerate, chi gong is just as beneficial as yoga and tai chi, and is particularly relevant if you already have health problems. (See the Resources section for tai chi and chi gong contacts.)

Because a relaxed body and calm mind are so essential in cancer prevention, these Eastern forms of exercise are strongly recommended. However, a very important role still exists for good old-fashioned aerobic exercise such as running, swimming, cycling, and other sports. It is particularly good for you to get some of your aerobic exercise in the fresh air. The ideal would be to attend a weekly class of yoga, tai chi, or chi gong, and then to practice at least fifteen to twenty minutes of daily stretching or exercising in one of these disciplines at home. Complement this with one or two sessions of aerobic exercise per week, one of which is outdoors, provided, of course, you can exercise in a nonpolluted location (it is better to jog in a gym than along a road with heavy traffic).

In addition, try to walk or to ride your bike whenever you can rather than taking the car, and make sure you do some form of stretching every day. If you cannot perform yoga, tai chi, or chi gong techniques, carry out your own stretch routine. Stretch your arms above your head to extend your spine, do side bends to stretch your waist, and incorporate a spinal twist. As well as helping to prevent cancer, regular stretching will make a huge difference in your posture, vitality, and well-being, not to mention your looks. If you are uninterested in trying Eastern exercise, the next best thing is to swim regularly. Swimming exercises every part of the body, and its avoidance of stress on the joints makes it relaxing.

If you have difficulties with mobility and all of this seems out of reach, think again—it is possible to perform many yoga stretches while sitting in a chair or even in bed. Tapes are available to help you adapt yoga to your own physical state (see the Resources section). Additionally, hydrotherapy exercise classes are offered at many swimming pools for those who are limited physically. In fact, if your mobility is limited, it is even more important to try to get some form of physical exercise. If this is not possible, consider getting a weekly massage. A good massage therapist can help shift toxins out of the body by a technique called lymph drainage (see the Resources section).

Dealing with Stress, Anxiety, and Overwork

Stress, anxiety, and overwork are usually connected to each other in a horrible, vicious cycle. If you feel anxious about money, work performance, or making a good impression on others in order to get a promotion or bonuses, affection, or sex, you are likely to push yourself harder and harder at work, at home, or in social situations. The resulting stress is exacerbated further if you are the sort of person who takes on more and more without thinking through the cost in terms of finance, time, energy, and personal compromise. If you are also a perfectionist or workaholic and have high integrity but poor self-esteem, the demands you make on yourself can become ridiculous.

Stress in the early stages is a form of excitement or a healthy response to a challenge or threat. In fact, in its early stages, stress can greatly improve performance. A healthy stress level can bring out the best in people, helping them to break through the inertia or laziness that makes them underachieve. However, the greater the anxiety, the pressure, and the fear of failure, the higher stress levels soar, to the point where people go beyond optimum performance. When this happens, they work harder and harder but achieve less and less. At this point there is serious risk of burnout. Individuals start displaying the telltale signs, such as inappropriate emotional reactions, bad decisions, and failure to meet deadlines, and they feel an ever-increasing sense of panic, despair, and helplessness as their situation grows further out of control. This stage is sometimes accompanied by physical exhaustion, which actually prevents people from working harder. But if their stamina is good, individuals will often respond to these feelings by trying to drive themselves even harder, until they are literally forced to stop by a mental breakdown or physical illness.

In Western society, high stress and anxiety levels are reaching epidemic proportions. A combination of factors—the cost of living; the complexity of the roles, demands, and expectations we all face; the tendency to drive ourselves hard—is putting our health and well-being at grave risk. And this is before we take into account the personal tragedy of discovering that we have managed to squeeze all the joy, fun, creativity, and, often, love out of life.

Various studies show that stress puts people at greater risk of cardiovascular disease, high blood pressure, heart attacks, and strokes. But what is not so clearly emphasized is the effect this kind of stress has on the immune system, predisposing us to cancer and infection at one extreme and allergic and autoimmune diseases at the other.

If you recognize that you are in a spiraling cycle of stress, you must take action immediately. This applies as much to people who are officially employed as to those who are not. Many people who are unemployed or who are at home taking care of small children get just as stressed as people with high-powered careers and important jobs. In fact, when stress is linked to power, the negative effects on health are not as great as when it is associated with powerlessness. Caring for sick relatives, elderly parents, or small children, with all the juggling of tasks and priorities this involves, combined with personal sacrifices, frustration, and lack of personal space and time to achieve your own goals can make people severely stressed. Indeed, any situation in which there are deep and complex conflicting emotions can trigger stress, in the same way that overactivity can.

Stress has two major components. One is so-called external stress, which comes from your environment and your relationship to it. This covers everything from the stress of heavy work deadlines, trying to drive across a busy city at rush hour, living or working in a hostile environment, getting married or divorced, losing a loved one, or going on vacation, to the need to bring home enough money to pay the bills each month.

The second component is internal stress. This is stress that arises as a result of your relationship with yourself. Most people are fairly conscious of the first form of stress, but are largely unconscious of the ways they stress themselves. Because internal stress tends to mirror our early life experiences and upbringing, our relationship with ourselves often reflects the type of relationship we had with key adults in our childhood. For example, if you had a harsh, critical, judgmental parent, chances are you have adopted these qualities in your own personality and in your relationship with yourself. If so, you very likely criticize yourself mercilessly, and push yourself harder and harder to achieve the kinds of results this harsh parent would have found acceptable.

Perhaps even more common are people who did not receive the love and affection they needed. They stress themselves interminably, trying to win love and approval from others, jumping through all kinds of hoops in order to do this. In fact, it is more often than not our relationship with ourselves and our past history that determines the level of *external* stress we put ourselves through. Where we live, how we work, and the demands we make on ourselves and others frequently come from our underlying sense of who we are and what we should be doing with our lives. For example, if you were brought up in affluent surroundings, had a private-school education, and enjoyed international travel and designer clothes, you are likely to put immense pressure on yourself to keep up this type of lifestyle. To this extent, many of us are "victims" of a large number of relatively unconscious forces that push us into lifestyles that make us miserable. The whole question of our relationship with ourself—and how to change it—will be addressed in Chapter 5. Meanwhile, the remainder of this chapter focuses on how to become aware of your stress levels, and how to make practical changes to bring them under control.

Looking for Signs of Stress

Most of us know if we are stressed. We feel anxious, irritable, miserable, and pressured. Physical signs of stress include a rapid, racing heartbeat, palpitations (where the heart misses a beat or jumps around irregularly), shallow breathing, indigestion, diarrhea, or constipation (sometimes accompanied by hemorrhoids). As stress levels become severe, people become less effective in everything they do. Being ineffective may be difficult to own up to, but it is better if you can spot it before it is pointed out to you by others—especially at work.

At this point people often say, "I feel like I'm running as fast as I can, but I just can't keep up—in fact, I feel like I'm going backwards." This may be followed by feelings of despair, because they are facing collapse. With severe stress like this, it becomes impossible to distinguish between key tasks and trivia. People are often only able to deal with the tip of the iceberg—coping with what is immediately in front of them, answering phone calls and letters and the like—and failing to do any strategic thinking or planning to make sure life will run smoothly and efficiently.

Another alarming symptom of severe stress is "thought block," when midsentence you can't remember what you were talking about. Sometimes, when stress levels are really high, this can lead to full-blown panic attacks, when ordinary anxiety spirals into terror and people become so paralyzed by fear that it is impossible to think clearly. At this point, medical help is often required.

If you suffer from any of these symptoms or are driving colleagues or family members into stress through your behavior, it is extremely important to stop now and address these issues in order to help prevent cancer and other serious illnesses.

Reducing Stress Levels

The practical way of dealing with stress embraces two fundamental approaches. First, tackle the symptoms of stress through relaxation, exercise, and meditation. Learning how to meditate or relax will be described fully later in the chapter. (A healthy approach to exercise was covered earlier in the chapter, in the section "Exercise.") Second, reorganize your day, at home or at work, to remove any unnecessary sources of stress, prioritizing those activities that are absolutely necessary.

Nine times out of ten, reducing stress levels means simplifying your life: This means having to let things go. People who are stressed almost always have needs, commitments, and expectations that are beyond their ability to "deliver"—at work or financially or emotionally. Getting life so out of balance is nearly always a sign of displaced emotional need, combined with a sense that everything will be all right if only something can be achieved, sorted out, or bought.

When stress becomes severe, most people need a break of two to four weeks with support and therapeutic help in order to allow the body to rebalance itself. In this situation, it is wise to start a program of relaxation, counseling, and physical therapies such as massage, aromatherapy, reflexology, and spiritual healing in order to help equilibrium become reestablished. Counseling is usually necessary because stressed people tend to suppress emotion—indeed, it may be the case that emotion has caused the stress in the first place. Spiritual healing might be available on a pay-as-you're-able basis; it can be an invaluable source of support at these times. (See more about spiritual healing below, in the section "Achieving and Maintaining High Energy Levels" that starts on page 170.) If the above options are unavailable, alternatively try to let yourself sleep and rest as deeply as possible.

In extreme cases of stress and burnout, it is usually impossible to think clearly enough to reorganize your priorities and simplify your life. It is therefore wise not to even try until after an initial phase of rest and therapeutic input, when your stress levels have fallen. Part of the problem of stress is that people can no longer see the forest for the trees, which makes it very difficult to prioritize.

Once your stress levels have reduced, it is a good idea to sit down with either your family or your work team and discuss the problem. Without a doubt, if you are feeling stressed, those around you will be stressed too. By getting control of the situation, you will be doing everybody in your immediate circle a favor. At first, this might make you feel very vulnerable. But getting the support of your family or colleagues is ultimately a helpful and bonding process. Explain to everyone that you are making a radical reappraisal of the way you live your life. If you can get them on board before you start, you will meet far less resistance and may even experience some solidarity.

At work, you may have to seek the help of an external consultant to manage organizational stress or to see where you are losing efficiency and building stress into your system. You may also need to work with a mentor to learn new, more effective ways of running your working life. In your personal life, a stress or debt counselor may be needed to help you sort out your problems, priorities, and goals.

Be aware that this simplifying and letting-go process may involve disappointment and feelings of loss, as you give up things you have been struggling to achieve. However, you may discover in the long term that, paradoxically, as you *do* less you start to *achieve* more. This becomes clear when you start to meditate. When you establish a regular meditation routine, life becomes much easier, and things you have planned or visualized start coming to you— you no longer have to struggle all the time to *make* them happen. It is absolutely remarkable how, once you start to "get yourself out of the way," the underlying process of life can start to support you.

Overcoming Severe Stress

The golden rules for bringing severe stress under control are:

1. Take a good two- to six-week break from all normal activity. In addition, work out a stress-busting program of relaxation, massage, and exercise to lessen the grip of stress on your body, and counseling to unburden yourself emotionally. Do not start work or normal activity again until at least a week after all the physical and mental symptoms of stress have disappeared.

2. When preparing to go back to work, go through your calendar and cancel every engagement or meeting over the next six months that is not absolutely vital.

3. Once you are able to think clearly again, consider what your priorities are and how you spend your time. List all your regular commitments, both at home and at work, and calculate the percentage of your time you give to each area of your life:

   ❖ important relationships

   ❖ caring for dependent relatives or friends

   ❖ social life

   ❖ clubs or societies you belong to

   ❖ management of changes at home (e.g., moving, remodeling, getting divorced, weddings, bereavement)

   ❖ the activities of children or partners in which you are involved

   Remember also to include:

   ❖ time for rest, exercise, relaxation, and recreation

   ❖ time for work commitments

   ❖ unstructured time just for you

   When you have worked out the percentage of time you normally devote to each area, the figures may be quite eye opening, showing clearly where the imbalance is. Most people find that work takes up the majority of their time and energy and causes the most stress. The other major cause is usually looking after other people's needs. Probably the main reason that most people get stressed, though, is quite simply because they forget to set time aside for themselves. They allow no time for rest, recuperation, reflection, and creativity, or to process and digest what is happening in their life. Over time, the failure to take time to be nourished and find meaning in life makes people feel bored, unsatisfied, empty, and depressed. It is their need to fill this sense of emptiness and to make themselves feel better, that often causes people to use alcohol or drugs. Sometimes these difficult feelings cause people to give even more of themselves to others, which drains them still further.

4. Make a new list of priorities by reorganizing your first list, allocating the correct proportion of time to the key areas in your life.

The fundamental purpose or goal of this process is to enable you to become clear again about your core values and to radically simplify your life so that you bring the most energy you can to the areas that matter the most to you. The foundation to all of this is to take proper time for yourself: This should appear at the top of your new list. Ideally, time for yourself should include totally unstructured time, as well as time to relax, meditate, exercise, and seek help from support groups, counselors, or therapists. It should also include at least one creative activity. This may mean, for example, reviving an interest in art, music, literature, theatre, or dance. Creating unstructured time means leaving space for yourself each week just to putter, rest, reflect, or read. If you live with others, you must guard your private time fiercely, and get the people in your life to respect your special time alone. Your doing so may even encourage them to do the same.

Making time for yourself is a particularly helpful example to give children. Many adults program their children for stress in later life. They organize their children's lives without leaving any space or "down time" when they can be alone in their inner world. It then becomes increasingly hard for them to be on their own, which is why so many adults find it difficult to be on their own and to develop a sustaining inner life. It is important, therefore, to start right from the beginning with children, allowing them space and time to unfold in their own creative, inner-directed way.

Once you have penned in time for yourself as your number-one priority in your new schedule, you will probably need to let go of as many as 50 percent of all your other activities and projects. This may sound drastic, but half of the extra time you create by doing so will be for yourself, with the rest for doing properly the things you are committed to, without rushing or struggling. It will also leave room for the inevitable growth of your activities. You may eventually have to do another major pruning exercise.

At work, reducing your goals by 50 percent will take a great deal of clarity, courage, and discipline. But taking the stress off yourself in this way will allow you in the end to achieve far better results on the projects you are working on. If this is simply impossible in your job, it may well be time for a change or to seriously challenge your managers about your job description. Usually, however, we are the ones who make our jobs impossible, either by being too ambitious or unrealistic, or by being incapable of saying no.

To combat severe stress you may need to reevaluate your belief that "more is better." Many of us think that others will consider us virtuous or more lovable if we are high achieving. But the tendency to take on more and more responsibilities can also be seen as a form of greed. It may look virtuous or altruistic, but often it is driven, just like overeating, by an underlying hunger for more— more power, more money, or more recognition. These needs, in turn, ultimately stem from an emotional or spiritual hunger that can be filled in far less destructive ways if emotional and spiritual needs are properly met. To address these underlying needs, many people need counseling help.

If you suffer from stress that is extreme, it is still important to establish a stress-reduction program that involves a mixture of relaxation and self-help techniques alongside your normal work. You can then trim and reprioritize your home, work, and social activities as discussed above, making sure to allow plenty of time for you.

Sleep, Rest, and Relaxation

To become really healthy and to avoid cancer, it is vital to address the need for proper sleep, rest, and relaxation. Sometimes, I like to think of life as being like an infinity sign, imagining that we move outward on one loop of the sign into activity, arousal, and achievement; then flow back again on an equal and opposite loop into rest, relaxation, letting go, and regeneration.

Sleep and Rest

Ayurveda is an ancient traditional system of Indian medicine that blends together yoga and herbal and nutritional medicine. It emphasizes our need to be in harmony with both the natural world and our own personal nature if we are to be truly healthy. Ayurvedic physicians believe that the body goes through a series of six four-hour cycles every day that start at 2:00, 6:00, and 10:00 A.M., and 2:00, 6:00, and 10:00 P.M. At 10:00 P.M., the end of the evening cycle, we naturally feel sleepy and ready to rest. However, if we resist this urge and stay up, we go into a new, more fiery type of energy cycle that may keep us up late into the night. This means, in effect, that if we then need to get up early to work or take care of children, we are burning the candle at both ends and failing to get the restorative rest and sleep we need.

Many people feel naturally sleepy around 9:30 to 10:00 P.M. and could easily go to bed then, but they override those feelings in order to achieve more and in an attempt to have more relaxation time. In the Ayurvedic system, the best time to get up is at daybreak, soon after 6:00 A.M. Try to get your life more in harmony with these natural cycles of the body. Try also to make the cutoff point for all work-related activity the moment you walk through the door at home after work. If this is not possible, then make an absolute deadline of about 8:00 P.M., after which all time is spent relaxing and nourishing yourself in creative ways.

Start going to bed or settling down around 10:00 P.M.—whether this is to read, meditate, reflect, write in a journal, or make love. All these things will deepen your connection with yourself and your loved ones. Make sure this gentle time is absolutely sacrosanct in your home life. Achieving this balance will make your life instantly richer and far healthier. Your immune system and tissue functioning will recover, and the risk of cancer will diminish greatly.

Relaxation

Relaxing is something many of us either have forgotten how to do or never knew how to do in the first place. We have become used to feelings of pressure, anxiety, and insecurity, and as a result many people are very tense. As a doctor, when I ask people if they are able to relax, they often say, "Yes, I can relax really easily. All I have to do is close my eyes and I fall asleep right away." But they do not realize that sleep is not the same as relaxation.

In fact, people who go to sleep tense or anxious often wake up just as anxious, because the body continues to make the stress chemicals adrenaline, noradrenaline, and cortisol throughout the night. Consequently, people who go to sleep anxious often have anxious dreams, which can leave them feeling ragged and exhausted the next day.

If sleep comes the instant you close your eyes, it may mean you are exhausted, often because of stress. If all this sounds familiar, you need to get yourself properly relaxed, either by consulting a relaxation therapist, yoga teacher, massage therapist, or healer, or by using a relaxation tape. These practices will allow you to experience what it feels like to be deeply relaxed, and will show you what to aim for when doing relaxation exercises on your own.

Relaxation removes the effects of stress and fear from the body and helps the mind unwind. When you prepare to do a relaxation exercise—with a relaxation therapist or on your own—first make yourself really comfortable and ensure that you are not going to be disturbed. Loosen tight clothing, remove shoes, glasses, or tight jewelry, and make sure you can get into a comfortable reclined position, preferably with your feet level with or slightly above your head. At first, it is best not to do relaxation exercises on your bed because you will probably fall asleep. You may also find that as you relax you will feel chilly, so cover yourself with a light blanket. Consider unplugging the telephone. Put a "Do Not Disturb" sign on your door, or ask others not to interrupt you for at least half an hour.

Now, settle into position—sitting on a chair or sofa, or lying on the floor—and allow yourself to feel very heavy, as if you have completely let go. A good relaxation therapist, teacher, or tape will usually invite you to consciously "unplug" yourself from all your normal activities so that you can switch off completely for the next fifteen or twenty minutes.

Start the relaxation exercise by breathing in deeply, as if right from the soles of your feet; then breathe out, making an audible sighing sound as you do. Do this three times. This signals the body to let go. Thereafter, focus your attention on breathing, allowing the breath to deepen and the whole breathing pattern to relax. Once you reach a safe, cocooned space, mentally go through each area of your body, consciously releasing tension as you do so. Most people start at the top of the head and work downward. Begin with the scalp, allowing it to relax and let go. Then go one by one to the forehead, eyes, cheeks, mouth, tongue, jaw, and throat, releasing any tension you encounter.

Some people prefer to tense each area of the body as they come to it, actively squeezing the muscles tightly and then relaxing them. They find this makes it easier to focus on specific areas. With either technique, attention then goes to the neck, shoulders, arms, and chest. In the chest area, pay particular attention to the rib cage, allowing it to relax so that breathing can become deeper. Also pay special attention to the abdomen, where an enormous amount of tension and anxiety can be held in the solar plexus and surrounding musculature. Then move to the hips, pelvis, thighs, knees, calves, ankles, and feet.

Theoretically, by the time you get to the tips of the toes, your whole body should be completely soft and relaxed. But in reality, while you are learning the technique, by the time you get to your toes the head and shoulders may have tensed up again. It may be worth repeating the whole exercise two or three times until you learn to let go fully throughout the entire body.

Once you achieve deep relaxation, either your body will feel very heavy or you will hardly be able to feel it at all. Our sense of position comes from nerve endings in the joints and balance receptors in the middle ear. If there is no movement in the body at all, as in a deep state of relaxation, we may temporarily lose the ability to tell where our body is. In this state, breathing should be slow and shallow and the heart rate will slow down. In stark contrast, when someone is stressed and mentally agitated, the heart rate is rapid, possibly with palpitations, muscles are tense, and breathing is irregular. When they are very anxious, people may even hold their breath.

Once you have experienced deep relaxation and have learned to achieve this state on your own, you can practice relaxing for twenty minutes a day at home, or perhaps during a break at work. As people get more experienced at relaxing, they can stay relaxed for much longer. Many of us put far too much energy and effort into everything we do, getting more and more tense as we go along. When you have mastered relaxation, check every hour or so to see how much you have tensed up again. Consciously release any tension in your shoulders, jaw, and stomach, and return your breathing to a normal, deep, slow rate. Over time, a relaxed state will become the norm, and feeling tense will become odd. Teach yourself the "magic of minimal effort": Put only the minimum amount of effort required into all you do. You will soon find that you are doing less but achieving more.

Achieving and Maintaining High Energy Levels

The importance of maintaining high energy levels and vitality was explained earlier, in the section "The Energy Model of Health." Eating well, exercising, resting, and relaxing all raise energy levels. But if you think your energy has dropped below the critical 30 percent level, it is time to lift it again through either spiritual healing or the energy medicines—shiatsu, acupuncture, and homeopathy.

Spiritual Healing

If you have never tried spiritual healing or are skeptical, I urge you to give it a chance and try it for yourself. You do not need to be religious or to have faith for spiritual healing to work.

During a healing process, the healer meditates or prays for your healing; then, by placing his or her hands close to your body, he or she becomes an "energy channel." This means that the healer becomes a conduit for energy from higher sources—either a divine power or the life force of nature or however you want to imagine it. It is impossible to say scientifically how this happens, but it quite definitely does. The resulting feeling is extremely nourishing and uplifting both for the one being healed and for the healer.

Those who have experienced healing describe quite a range of experiences. Frequently, individuals report that the healer's hands felt either very hot or very cold. When healing was given with the eyes closed, people report having seen colors or light in their mind's eye. For others, the experience can be emotionally releasing—experienced either as feeling suddenly safe or "held" enough to let go, or as a distinct sense of higher love that is very moving in a joyful way. By contrast, some people report a great quietening of their emotions with a growing sense of deep peace and relaxation. Others experience nothing at all at the time of their healing. However, whether or not this is the case, almost everyone who persists with regular spiritual healing feels a great improvement in their energy levels and ability to tackle their situation positively. Once they have tried healing, even people who were initially suspicious cannot deny that it is a lovely experience and that the effects make a real difference. After witnessing this process with cancer patients, I picture it this way: Initially, they are like boats in a harbor when the tide has gone out, completely grounded and unable to make a move in any direction. Once the energy flows back into them as a result of the healing, it is like the tide is in again. They are potent, able to move, make choices, and set off in a new, more meaningful direction.

The beauty of spiritual healing is that you do not have to think, talk, or do any work. The only requirement is that you be receptive to the healing energy. It is a bit like lying back and enjoying the sun or soaking in a warm bath. What proves hard for many people is the idea of letting go and receiving from others. Such an admission of our vulnerability is often difficult to make. Indeed, many people in a depleted energy state try very hard to keep everything together, instead of resting and regenerating. If your energy levels have fallen very low, spiritual healing may be necessary two or three times a week until they rise to the point where you can begin to help yourself with yoga, tai chi, meditation, relaxation, and exercise.

If you cannot get to a healer, you could try absent healing. To locate a healer in your area, or to ask for absent healing, contact the UK-based National Federation of Spiritual Healers, the World Light Center, or www.silentunity.com (see the Resources section).

The Energy Medicines: Shiatsu, Acupuncture, and Homeopathy

Shiatsu and acupuncture are the traditional medicines of Japan and China respectively. In both systems, one's energy state is diagnosed by reading energy pulses. In acupuncture, pulses are taken at the wrist; in shiatsu they are taken in the abdomen or *hara*. With this information, a rebalancing of the body's energy can be carried out. In acupuncture this is done with needles; in shiatsu it is done with pressure from the fingers, hands, or even elbows at pressure points throughout the body.

In the East it is said that traditionally people paid their acupuncturists while they were well and stopped paying if they became sick. For centuries these systems of medicine have been used primarily for prevention rather than treatment. It is an extremely useful attitude and behavior for us in the West to adopt. An acupuncturist or shiatsu practitioner can quickly tell what the underlying state of your energy is. You may need several sessions to get into a good state of balance, and once this has been achieved you may need to go monthly or every six weeks in order to maintain a high energy state and help prevent cancer.

Like shiatsu and acupuncture, homeopathy raises and balances the vital force, but it is done through remedies given in tablet form, which interact with our own energy to optimize our state of health and vitality. Homeopathy was founded by Samuel Hahneman, circa 1750, in Germany. He noted that the same substances that caused symptoms of illness in the well could alleviate those same symptoms in the well. Astonishingly, he then discovered that their power to do so increased with their dilution—the highest potency remedies being the most dilute. From there he went on to discover "constitutional remedies" that fit with the different characteristics and symptom patterns seen in distinct types of people. He found that when patients were given the correct constitutional remedy, many symptoms of illness could be treated simultaneously with a marked improvement in health. In present times, homeopathy can still be used in both ways. It is used quite commonly to help control the symptoms of cancer and the side effects of its treatment, but for preventive purposes the best results come from being treated systemically with a constitutional remedy. This is analogous to the difference between acupuncture being used for pain relief or to help with the cessation of smoking versus its use in the traditional way for overall rebalancing of the bodies "chi"/vitality and general health. In homeopathy the chi is referred to as the vital force.

Working with Your Energy

For the long term, the way to achieve optimum health and high energy levels is to be aware of what you do with your energy—how you spend it and how you regain it. Many people's energy levels resemble a seriously overdrawn bank balance—they expend energy recklessly without a thought as to how they will replenish it. In fact, a tendency to overspend money often goes hand in hand with a tendency to overexpend energy. Overspending, like overeating, may be a compensation for emptiness inside, caused by failing to nourish ourselves emotionally and spiritually. Others find themselves depleted in energy because they simply don't have adequate support to cope with their commitments to a partner, children, elderly relatives, work, and home life.

Begin to look at where you are expending or even hemorrhaging vital energy. Many of us spend vast amounts of energy getting caught up in the affairs of others or battling our way through the stores when they are crowded. We try to sustain crazy social or work lives and remain involved in draining relationships. Although we don't necessarily realize it, we may live or work in a place that drains our energy. Some people and places are like energy "black holes"—even a telephone call with someone like this can leave us depleted. Or we may lose energy, as mentioned earlier, simply by putting too much energy into everything we do.

Some people are more energy sensitive than others, but they are so tuned in to the energy of others that they lose track of how they feel themselves. These energy-sensitive people can become "symptom carriers" for their family or close friends since they are often empathic types. They tend to soak up difficult, unharmonious energies around them in an unconscious attempt to equilibrate and harmonize the atmosphere. Such people become particularly compromised if they fail to make space and time for themselves. If this describes you, make extra sure you spend plenty of time both on your own and around healthy energy. Learn to recognize people, places, and activities that enhance your energy levels. People often say that their energy levels are raised dramatically by trips to the country, gardens, forests, the desert; by beauty, music, and meditation; or simply by spending time alone either being still or in creative activity.

Once you start to think about it, you will begin to recognize exactly what feeds and drains your energy levels. You may find you are being propped up by the energy of another, perhaps because you are failing to take responsibility for building your own energy levels. It is important to change this pattern and raise your energy levels in a healthier way.

Make a list of the things that feed and drain your energy. You could even create a balance sheet and compare the debit and credit elements of your energy account. If it is clear that you are pouring your precious energy into nonproductive areas, gradually start to eliminate the depleting activities and replace them with things that lift your energy. This practice will overlap with your efforts to reduce stress, because cutting down on planned activities, whether in your social or your work life, will also have a big effect on energy levels. But the things that drain energy are different from stress: Certain situations or people, for example, can take a lot of your energy without your necessarily giving them much time. If, along with reprioritizing your time, you also start to avoid draining phone calls, difficult people, unnecessary shopping trips, and other nonproductive behavior, replacing all this "doing" with simply "being," your energy levels will rise dramatically.

Care must be taken over the issue of energy and exercise. Sometimes, exercising hard when you have little energy can reduce energy levels further. However, exercising when your energy levels are beginning to rise will strengthen you and raise your energy even more. It is a question of being aware of the effect exercise has on your energy levels. This is also relevant to what has been said about resting—once you are more aware of what is going on with your underlying energy, you will stop overriding the signals from your body that indicate you are tired and will instead listen to your body and rest appropriately.

As energy levels rise you will experience an enhanced sense of intuition and connection with life, more synchronicity or meaningful coincidences, and heightened telepathic ability. In other words, as energy levels rise, so does our state of consciousness. Most importantly, people with an abundance of energy are happier, more confident and in control, and more able to live meaningful, creative lives.

Cancer is much less likely to develop when the body is in a high-energy state. It has been shown that in those with higher energy, immune and enzyme activity increases at the cellular level. High energy literally wakes up the body's tissues and defense mechanisms. This makes cell nuclei far less likely to mutate, and if they do, they are quickly picked up and eradicated from the body.

Being excited, enthusiastic, and passionate about life has the most profound effect on energy and vitality. When we suddenly find love, become fully expressed in our work, or open the door to our spirituality, energy levels can jump right off the graph.

Calming Your Mind with Meditation

When Zoe Lindgren was diagnosed with breast cancer, she was pregnant with her second child. Doctors advised her to terminate the pregnancy. But Zoe, who was thirty-one at the time, refused. Six months into the pregnancy, she had a lumpectomy to remove the cancerous growth, and after her daughter was born she underwent radiation.

As soon as Zoe was diagnosed with cancer, she went to the Bristol Cancer Help Centre. Because she had cared for her mother with cancer, she was already aware of the Centre's work. The main change she made at this point was to become a vegetarian.

Two years later, in 1991, she was diagnosed with cancer again, but this time it was in her lungs and lymph system. Zoe was told that even with chemotherapy she had only a maximum of eighteen months to live. While undergoing chemotherapy she felt at her lowest ebb, and it became of paramount importance to her that she regain control of what was a very out-of-control situation. She was determined not to become a victim and wanted to make the experience as positive as she could. After four of her six scheduled chemotherapy sessions, she could take no more. She ended conventional medicine and turned instead to complementary therapies to help her confront her illness, mental state, and lifestyle.

Zoe recognized immediately that the biggest problem she had to tackle was her pressure-filled lifestyle and the stress levels she endured as a successful architect. She knew that if her body was to survive, it was vital to calm her mind, so she embarked on a concentrated program of mind/body techniques, favoring particularly meditation and visualization. At first she found the new regimen an uphill struggle. But with the guidance and support of the Bristol Cancer Help Centre, she was able to master the techniques. She also underwent acupuncture, homeopathy, spiritual healing, and reflexology, and found emotional support from her husband, Andy. She learned through counseling about being nonjudgmental, about how to look at the positive side of things, and about the harmful effects on the body of a negative self-image.

But the most important thing of all, she feels, was her decision to leave behind her life in the fast lane to live in a forest in Wales. Since making this move, Zoe has become a completely different woman. The combination of her peaceful home, daily meditations, and healthy diet has turned her into a radiant picture of health, and she now positively emanates health, well-being, and tranquillity.

Ten years later, at forty-three, Zoe is still cancer-free, and is working part-time as a reflexologist. While she is sure the chemotherapy and tamoxifen she took in 1991 "doused the fire" of the disease, she has outlived her prognosis by years and has clearly achieved a most remarkable recovery. She has done everything in her power to prevent the disease from recurring and has achieved an absolutely outstanding stabilization of her condition.

Zoe now enjoys a much better quality of life than ever before; she feels her greatest achievement has been the development of inner strength and peace of mind. Her success is an enormous testimony to the power of the holistic approach to health and is a fitting reward for all the hard work she has put into her recovery process. Zoe's story clearly demonstrates the need, above all others, to reduce our stress levels and achieve inner peace if we want to get well and stay well.

The single most beneficial thing you can do to revolutionize your health is to start meditating. This will make every other aspect of your life easier. As you become calmer with a clearer state of mind, your energy levels will quickly rise. Resistance and inertia will melt away, and you will find it easier to put all other aspects of life on a healthier footing. Neuroses will lose their grip, and you will once again be able to see the forest for the trees.

It is important to say here that learning to meditate does not involve becoming part of a sect or taking up a religion. You can meditate in a religious context, within Buddhism, say, but it is equally possible to meditate without any religion or belief system at all.

Meditation involves calming the mind so that you can experience pure consciousness and the connection between your consciousness and all that surrounds you. Many people go through life without ever experiencing this clear state of mind. Instead, they are preoccupied with what goes on in their minds and with their sense of separation from everything and everybody. Many of us believe that we *are* our thoughts, feelings, sensations, and emotions, but actually these things are the *contents* of our consciousness rather than our consciousness itself.

When we learn how to still our minds and get untangled from the contents of consciousness, we discover that the natural underlying state of our consciousness is one of bliss. This is why all the religious texts of the world say that the kingdom of heaven is within. As soon as this still and open state of mind is discovered, people quickly realize that it feels better than much of the external stimulation they seek. As a result, their continual quest for external satisfaction diminishes and their inner state becomes greatly enriched. Although people still need to fulfill their potential in life, this is likely to happen in a far more gentle, wholesome, and satisfying manner.

Psychologically, the great benefit of meditation is that emotions begin to settle and people become more sensitive to their own inner voice of wisdom. This wise part of ourselves will often know exactly what we need or don't need in any given situation. As people base their lives more and more on the wisdom of this inner-knowing or higher self, a lot of problems and neurotic behavior will simply dissolve away.

On a physiological level, the chaotic beta waves associated with intense mental activity and stress are replaced with gentler alpha waves. At deeper levels of meditation these can be replaced by very slow delta or even theta waves. When this happens, the neuropeptide cocktail in the body is changed entirely, and tissues and cells begin to function optimally.

All committed meditators report a wonderfully enhanced sense of living in harmony with nature, and feel supported by life rather than constantly struggling against it. Their sense of separation and isolation is diminished, eventually replaced with a wonderful sense of connection to life and a feeling of being part of the whole. However, many people are addicted to chaos and emotional drama and will resist attempts to quiet down emotionally. But once the addiction to pain and emotional drama is replaced with real joy, a much deeper and more satisfying sense of emotional fulfillment and pleasure can be attained.

In relation to cancer, meditation alone has been shown to heal the disease. This is demonstrated by the work in Australia of Ainsley Mearess, who took people with cancer into prolonged states of meditation. In many cases the deep calming and reactivation of the immune system led to quite extraordinary remission and healing—powerful proof of the connection between mind and body. There are some who say the cellular chaos of cancer is a reflection of our mental and emotional chaos. And it may be that until we sort out our collective fear and disharmony, we will never be able to eradicate cancer. I am sure there is a great deal of truth in this, because of the profound effects of our state of mind on tissue functioning. That is why I believe meditation holds the most potential for turning around our susceptibility to cancer.

Learning Meditation

There are many ways to learn meditation. The practice always involves focusing attention on a single thing until the mind becomes so still that it transcends even that focus. This can be a sound—or *mantra* as it is called in yogic practice—repeated in your head. It can be a visual object or picture such as a mandala—an image that draws your focus to its center. Or you can keep your attention fixed on the flow of your breathing. Other forms of meditation involve focusing on loving feelings in your heart and on generating feelings of love for yourself and the rest of humanity and the world. Some traditions focus on the sensation of the skin. This technique is often used in Vipassana meditation.

The best-known school of meditation, using a mantra technique, is transcendental meditation (TM); this is a highly effective way of learning the skill. Focusing on the breath is often associated with yogic and Buddhist practices; teachers for these techniques can be found through the Friends of the Western Buddhist Order as well as other schools of meditation (see the Resources section).

For many of us, learning to meditate is difficult because we have busy minds and have never learned how to still them. To master the technique, one must commit to adequate training and regular practice. Joining a regular meditation class or group is highly recommended until you are able to meditate for at least twenty minutes a day at home by yourself. Initially, meditating in a group will make the practice far easier, for the stillness and peace generated by the group will be contagious. Whatever else you do as a result of reading this book, I urge you most strongly to develop a meditation practice. This will undoubtedly unlock your ability to take the right steps toward health, well-being, and fulfillment in all areas of your life.

5

❖❖❖

Working with the
Mind/Body/Spirit Connection

The most profound difference you can make in your health is to
attend to the underlying state of your spirit. You can do this
directly through meditation, but you can also do it by unburdening
your spirit and moving toward a lifestyle that expresses and nour-
ishes you. Doing so will enable you to become truly well, from the
inside out. When you are at peace with yourself, living authenti-
cally, fully engaged with life in a meaningful and exciting way, the
reverberations of this extremely wholesome feeling will affect the
way every tissue and cell of your body functions, and you will
become healthy and alive.

Here are two good examples of the changes in health that can
occur when people start to live in ways that are true to themselves.
The first concerns a patient of the brilliant dermatologist Dr. Ann
McGuire, who became renowned for her unique approach to skin
problems, which involves working with the mind/body connection. The basic premise of her work holds that the skin is the mirror of the psyche. One time, at the end of a long, hard day in the
clinic, a man came in who had suffered from severe psoriasis for
many years. He had come expecting an in-depth exploration of the
emotional side of his skin problem. But instead he found an irritable, tired Ann who had simply run out of steam.

When he asked the doctor what was wrong with him, she replied, "It's quite simple—you are in the wrong place, at the wrong time, doing the wrong thing with your life." With this she closed his file and told him she could give him no more time. Later, she felt dreadful about having treated this poor man so dismissively, and was quite worried about the repercussions she might have to face. So when she saw his name on her patient list a few months later, she was sure he was going to be extremely angry with her. But this couldn't have been farther from the truth. He bounded into the room and practically kissed her! She quickly realized that his psoriasis had disappeared altogether. She asked him what on earth had happened.

> He replied, "Well, of course, you were completely right—I was in the wrong place, at the wrong time, doing the wrong thing with my life. For twenty years, I had been farming and slaughtering animals for meat. Running the slaughterhouse had actually been distressing me deeply. Over the years I became more and more revolted by the whole process, but I was unable to face getting rid of my farm and business and starting over in a new direction. When you said what you said, the whole thing came into focus for me and that same afternoon I put my business on the market. It sold within a month, and I am now in the process of turning my land over to crop farming. The minute I made the decision, it was as if a huge weight had been lifted off my shoulders. The relief was immense, and almost immediately the psoriasis started to shift. Now, for the first time in years, my skin is clear!"

From having started the consultation a very worried woman, Ann ended up celebrating with this man the powerful shift he had made in his life and health.

The second illustration comes from the area of cancer medicine, and is a good example of the work of Dr. Lawrence LeShan, one of the founders of the holistic health and mind/body medicine movement. Larry worked with cancer patients for many years, helping them get their lives on track in order to heal their disease. In this case his patient was a friend named Peter who was very ill with a serious pancreatic tumor. He had been told he had just weeks to live. Peter was in the hospital when Larry saw him, jaundiced and hooked up to an IV drip, looking pretty ghastly and feeling extremely depressed.

Larry started the conversation in his normal way, asking Peter what it was in life that really excited and motivated him. Knowing Larry well, Peter replied, "For goodness sake, Larry—can't you see I'm dying! This is no time to talk about what turns me on!" But Larry gently persisted, and after an hour or so ascertained that Peter's true passion was sculpture. However, the profession he had ended up following all his life, due to parental pressure, was architecture.

He had been a good and successful architect, but had never felt truly excited by his work. Larry asked him where, in an ideal world, he would have liked to study sculpture. Peter said, "Florence, of course!" Mischievously, taking a gamble, Larry said, "If I showed up here with a ticket to Florence and an opportunity to study sculpture there, would you take it?" Peter sat bolt upright and said, "Of course I would! What have I got to lose? I'm just sitting here waiting to die." This was all the encouragement Larry needed. He went off and with Peter's family arranged to get a plane ticket, and he found a sculpting course that was starting shortly in Florence.

Within a week Peter found himself in Florence, where he set up a small studio. He was weak, but his excitement and sense of anticipation were immense. He not only started and completed the six-month sculpting course, but also fell in love. He went on to enjoy an absolutely enchanting two years there, exploring his new relationship, his life passion of sculpting, and the wonderful museums and buildings of the city. At the end of this two years, he was called back to America on family business. Within three months of leaving Italy, his cancer returned with a vengeance. Three weeks later he died peacefully at home.

Peter died a very happy, grateful, and satisfied man. He had allowed his spirit to fly free for two glorious years, and as tough as it was to surrender to death after having known such sweetness, he was able to let go gracefully in the knowledge that, even if only for two years, he had been fully alive.

In the first of these cases, it was the release from terrible inner conflict that allowed the physical healing to occur. In the second, it was only when Peter became fully authentic and truly expressed himself that his immune system kicked in and stabilized the tumor. These cases illustrate just how profound the connection is between mind, body, and spirit, and how crucial it is to attend to our state of happiness and fulfillment if we really want to be well and to prevent cancer.

ATTENDING TO THE STATE OF YOUR SPIRIT

Attending to your spirit involves three main phases. The first is the *unburdening* phase. You need to unburden yourself of:

- ❖ emotions you have been carrying for a long time
- ❖ disabling attitudes or limiting beliefs that you picked up earlier in life
- ❖ roles you play or personas you project that do not represent who you really are
- ❖ dominating presences or forces in your life

The second phase involves *discovering who you really are.* This whole process could be described as becoming true to yourself. It entails:

- ❖ eliciting your core values in life (particularly what gives your life purpose or meaning)
- ❖ finding ways to express yourself in the world (with respect to your job, the environment in which you live, the relationships you choose, your sexuality, and so on, as well as the more obvious outlets you may have for your creative and physical energies, such as hobbies and sports you enjoy)

In essence, this step is all about you—the unique being that you are—becoming enabled and empowered to reach your full potential. It has absolutely nothing to do with competition with others; it is about allowing yourself to flourish and grow and to express your true nature, irrespective of anyone else.

The third area is attending to your spiritual nourishment. This may be through:

❖ beauty, art, or fine music

❖ religion

❖ meditation

❖ spiritual retreats

❖ developing your personal spirituality

❖ dedicated service to others

❖ sharing the spontaneous fun and creativity of children

❖ creative activity

❖ giving and receiving love

The ability to do any of these steps is based first and foremost on being prepared to develop a healthy relationship with yourself.

DEVELOPING A HEALTHY RELATIONSHIP WITH YOURSELF

If you are already able to take care of yourself well, the advice given here does not apply to you. Sadly, however, many of us fail to do this. We often appear at the bottom of our own list of people and things we're responsible for. As I've said before, some of us take far better care of our cars and our homes than we do of ourselves; we're careful to get our cars serviced regularly and keep our houses clean and well maintained. Perhaps if, like their cars, people were forced to undergo yearly inspections, they would neglect themselves less.

By answering the following questions, you will get a basic idea of what your relationship with yourself is like.

❖ Do you eat properly?

❖ Do you get enough sleep?

❖ Do you exercise regularly?

❖ Do you walk away from abusive relationships?

❖ Do you maintain your appearance?

❖ Do you stay out of debt?

❖ Do you refrain from abusing or harming yourself physically and mentally?

❖ Do you believe you are valuable?

❖ Do you believe you deserve attention, love, money, and nice possessions?

❖ Do you believe you are lovable?

❖ Are you able to spend time alone?

❖ Do you give yourself time for rest and recuperation?

And most important of all:

❖ Do you love, or even like, yourself?

If most of the answers to these questions are yes, your relationship with yourself is in pretty good shape. But if you came up with a lot of no answers, your relationship with yourself could probably stand some improvement. People who lack a good relationship with themselves and who fail to value themselves properly have low self-esteem. Under such conditions, people are unlikely to establish, let alone maintain, activities that allow them to fulfill themselves, and will find it difficult to implement any of the advice in this book. So, the first step in your resurrection and cancer-prevention program is to go about changing your relationship with yourself.

The relationship we have with ourselves usually resembles the relationship we had with our parents, or other significant adults, in childhood. If we were loved, cherished, nurtured, and encouraged, we will probably be good at doing this for ourselves. If, on the other hand, we were neglected, criticized, abandoned, abused, or shown very little encouragement or affection, this is also likely to be the way we will treat ourselves. If necessary, it is possible to change your relationship with yourself and to begin treating yourself well. More often than not, this requires the experience of a new kind of nurturing relationship with another person to reset the template. This is where counseling, psychotherapy, spiritual healing, and complementary therapies that employ touch can be extremely helpful.

All these emotional and physical therapies are based on treating the client with what is known as unconditional positive regard. This means the relationship is based on nonjudgmental lovingkindness, and care and concern for the client. All holistic therapies have at their root the aim of enabling you to develop this sort of relationship with yourself, so that when the period of therapy is over you can continue the nurturing process yourself. Once a caring relationship has been modeled for you, you will be able, bit by bit, to take over and start giving yourself what you really need.

If you feel your self-esteem is very low, you should probably go for counseling or psychotherapy. It is important to have an introductory meeting to make sure the therapist is suitable for you, rather than the other way round. If the experience is to build your self-esteem and confidence, you must feel entirely comfortable with this person and feel that he or she has genuine warmth toward you. Don't hesitate to meet with two or three therapists before you make your choice.

If you think you can build a new relationship with yourself without this kind of help, the golden rules are:

1. Learn to put yourself at the top of the list of people to take care of. When you look after yourself well, you are in better shape to care for others and will be giving them a terrific model to follow and apply in their own lives. You will also

enjoy a much healthier relationship with your partner. When you are able to care for yourself properly, you are far less needy and therefore far less likely to stay with an unsuitable partner, because you will be less dependent on the "crumbs from their table."

2. Get to know yourself and your needs well. Get used to tuning in to how you feel, and react appropriately. Be alert to your body's needs for food, sleep, sex, and exercise; your emotional needs for comfort, warmth, and support; and the needs of your soul or spirit for peace, space, or adventure.

3. Learn to express your feelings and to ask clearly for what you need—without getting upset if the answer is no. If this is hard for you, take a course in assertiveness to learn how to communicate your needs without fear and to accept a "no" without taking it as rejection.

4. Work through the questions at the beginning of this section, making sure you are taking care of yourself properly in all of these ways.

The above advice is mainly for people who are "other-centered," who cling to a negative self-image and poor self-esteem. But sometimes the reverse is the problem. If you have become rather self-centered, you need to learn to think and care more about the needs of others, as well as your own. Generally speaking, though, it is better to err on the side of being self-centered, because people are far more likely to take good care of themselves if they have a high opinion of themselves.

Having a good relationship with yourself can be described as being your own "good parent." You cease to be at the mercy of your needy, greedy, demanding, anarchic inner child and, instead, are able to give yourself what will nourish, sustain, and develop you throughout life. This means acquiring a more mature sense of what you really need, rather than always going for instant gratification or for what feels good at the time. This is not meant to diminish the value of spontaneity or of giving yourself treats, but it is important to know the difference between treats that will genuinely nurture you and those that will give you a boost now but cost you later.

In the transpersonal model of psychology, the different aspects of ourselves are seen as subpersonalities, whose needs have to be negotiated. As you become increasingly self-aware, many subpersonalities may emerge that you can recognize, work with, and care for.

Changing your relationship with yourself does not happen overnight. But as with everything else, embracing the intention to learn how to be gentler, more loving, more permissive, and more responsible toward yourself is a strong starting point. See if you can make this commitment to yourself now, before you read on about the practical steps to improve the state of your spirit. Once again, it may be a good idea to write down notes about the areas in which you wish to make changes in your life.

UNBURDENING THE SPIRIT

Letting Go of Emotions

Remember the holistic concept, "What the mind represses the body expresses"? Many people are simply too scared to express their feelings, but feelings have to go somewhere. A feeling produces chemical neuropeptides in the brain and body, and as feelings are expressed, these neuropeptides are discharged or metabolized, and equilibrium is restored. (Neuropeptides released in tears of rage, by the way, are completely different from those released in tears of grief or heartbreak.) Should these chemicals not be released, however, they become stuck in the body, causing physiological change. Dr. Candace Pert, who helped to discover neuropeptides, calls them "molecules of emotion" (see under "Books" in the Resources section).

It is useful to define our "feelings" as what we feel when something happens. When feelings remain unexpressed and turn into memories in the mind and body, they become emotions that may be retained for a long time. Sometimes people are comfortable expressing one kind of feeling but not others. For example, some of us find it easy to cry, but can't show our anger. For others, it is the reverse—they may erupt like a volcano but find it impossible to cry in public!

The most common feelings that people hang on to are grief, disappointment, bitterness, guilt, and anger. When these become lodged as emotions in the body, they can bear particular effects on different organs. For example, grief tends to affect the lungs and throat; anger affects the liver and gut; bitterness the pancreas; disappointment the kidneys; and guilt the nervous system. Though these are very broad generalizations, often observed through Eastern energy medicines, in practice, it is surprising how often these general rules hold true. All of the effects occur through PNI (psychoneuroimmunology), or mind/body mechanisms.

The emotions also have a major effect on the blood and immune systems. Stress and upset reduce the number of circulating immune cells and also make the immune cells less active, and decrease the amount of oxygen carried in the hemoglobin of red blood cells. If you are burdened with a lot of old emotion from upsets, losses, or frustrations suffered in the past, it is an extremely good idea, both for the health of your immune system and for your ultimate protection against cancer, to offload it. This can be done in many ways. The most common method is through counseling or psychotherapy, in which a person is taken directly to a particular emotional memory and allowed, in a variety of ways, to discharge the energy or emotion incurred at that time that they still hold onto or embody. In addition to counseling, there are also physiological methods that can be used. A professional massage or shiatsu—as well as powerful sex—often touch old emotions, which can then be expressed if support is present. Spiritual healing also unlocks emotional doors and promotes their release.

There are many trained professionals who can help you actively forgive and let go of old hurts or wounds. People often hang onto or even nurse old grievances, bearing grudges and resentments even against the dead. This is not a healthy way to live. Not only do we become clogged up with these harmful emotions, but part of our vital energy is trapped and inaccessible to us for living. Thus, some therapists and group counselors concentrate on the forgiveness approach. Many groups, classes, and opportunities exist for self-development work that focuses on the area of healing the past (see the Resources section at the back of the book).

Changing Difficult Attitudes and Limiting Beliefs

As well as forming the basis of our relationship with ourselves, early life is also the source of many of the underlying attitudes and beliefs that we hold about life and our abilities. When we are children we are very trusting and tend to believe what adults tell us. We are also equally affected by what they fail to tell us. If we get the message that we are not good enough, this will become our belief, and as adults we will tend to give up on even trying to get the things we want. If we do not get the attention and encouragement we need, we will believe we are unlovable and constantly strive for approval and attention.

If our environment as a child was hostile and abusive, we may view the world as a dangerous place and be constantly fearful and insecure (even if, to outsiders, our situation seems quite safe). If the parent figure in our life was harsh, critical, and judgmental, we may have become harsh and judgmental with ourselves. If we were told that children should be seen and not heard, we may find it difficult to be spontaneous or exuberant. If we were reprimanded every time we got angry or cried, then we probably now find it difficult to express emotion. If we discovered that the way to get attention was by being sexually provocative, we may be sexually manipulative as adults.

While these survival codes may work in childhood, when we are adults they can severely limit our pleasure and ability to fulfill our potential. Also, children can absorb a message that says they do not deserve good things, and so, when grown, would rather push good things away than endure the discomfort of receiving. People who overgive are often acting on this misconception carried over from their youth. Although they are very generous themselves, if you try to give them anything, they find it almost impossible to accept. Many of us continue to be influenced by a number of such limiting beliefs—that we don't deserve to have the love, money, power, or enjoyment we want and need—and as a result we live in a semidepressed state all our lives.

To turn this situation around, learn to recognize underlying attitudes that affect your behavior or curb your expectations, and replace them with healthier ones. This kind of work can be done with a transpersonal counselor (see the Resources section). Once you start looking, it is quite easy to unearth these beliefs. The way to replace them, first and foremost, is by challenging yourself every time you find one of these attitudes coming into play. You can also make a list of your unconstructive attitudes and limiting beliefs, and then make a second set of statements that reverse them. For example, if you first write "I am unlovable," take a second piece of paper and put down "I am lovable." If you believe "I do not deserve to be wealthy," write "I deserve wealth and abundance." Once you make a list of positive statements, you can use them as affirmations to repeat to yourself on a regular basis. You can also repeat and affirm them to yourself whenever you find that an old, limiting belief is "running you" in a given situation.

By doing this you will replace, over time, the negative messages of your upbringing with positive messages and beliefs. Eventually, you will be able to behave according to this new code rather than the old one. Although it is easier to do this work with a therapist, it is certainly possible to do it on your own, especially if you keep a journal and add to the list when you discover other ways that you limit or compromise yourself.

Shedding Unhelpful Roles and Personas

Our roles or personas in adult life are also an extension of the attitudes and beliefs we have adopted from childhood. For example, if the desire to win approval extends into your professional life, you may have chosen a well-respected role such as that of doctor, nurse, or minister. If you grew up believing that the world is a frightening place, you may have built your life around a need to be in control and thus have become a politician, teacher, policeman, or member of the armed forces. This is not to say that being a care-giver, politician, or policeman is not the perfect role in life for some people. It largely depends on whether you have taken on this role from strength or from weakness, from wholeness or from wounded-ness (your "shadow," as it is known in Jungian psychology). Ask yourself the following questions:

❖ Does my role genuinely reflect who I am, giving me excite-ment, life, and energy?

❖ Is my role driven by an underlying fear of some kind, or by a need for the secondary gains the role brings with it?

An example of a role or persona that is "shadow" driven would be a seemingly generous person who actually gives because of her own immense emptiness and need. By constantly and noticeably giving of herself, her time, or her money, she is really trying to show others how she would like to be treated herself, but is too scared to ask for. By overgiving she will become even more depleted and is ultimately likely to suffer from some form of burnout or depression. This has its foundations in the anger she feels inside at not being treated properly.

A useful way to look at your roles and personas is to think of them as subpersonalities. You can draw up a good "map" of your psyche by working with a therapist, by taking courses, or by think-ing about it on your own. You can learn which are your dominant subpersonalities and which hardly ever see the light of day. Some-times, one of the subpersonalities that has been submerged by the others can seem much more like the real you. Your true happiness may depend upon allowing this aspect of yourself to develop and come forward.

A good example of how this can work comes from a colleague of mine who had breast cancer. At the time, she was a school-teacher and "executive wife," hosting countless elaborate dinner parties for her husband's high-powered business associates. During a period of soul-searching after being diagnosed, she realized that none of these roles really matched her true self, and that, at heart, she was a "creative" who adored nature and natural medicine. Over time, she gradually withdrew from her former roles and allowed the gentler aspect of her personality to emerge. She now lives as a potter, organic gardener, and spiritual healer, and enjoys radiant good health twenty years after her initial diagnosis with breast cancer.

To identify your subpersonalities, allow yourself to go inside your psyche and conjure up in your mind's eye all the different aspects of yourself. Some will be obvious; others will be less obvious, but nonetheless very important. Maybe you are a combination of a bossy teacher, nature-loving gardener, opera singer, striptease artist, and Mother Teresa! Try to get a sense of which of your sub-personalities serve and express you well, and which give you the greatest energy. Compare these with the ones that compromise and drain you. If you are dissatisfied with certain aspects of your life, ask yourself whether it might be time to start moving toward expressing one of your less dominant qualities, one that would serve you better and make your life happier.

Getting Free of Dominant Presences or Forces

Sometimes people fail to express themselves effectively because somebody or something dominates them to such an extent that they don't know how they feel or what they want. We talk about being "possessed" by the dead, but it is also possible to be "possessed" or dominated by the living! People who were dominated as children by the emotional needs of their parents or siblings may live as adults in a state of constant reaction to the needs of other people. This can happen at home, at school, or at work—wherever they are confronted by a dominant character who manages to be the center of attention, manipulating others in the process. In partnerships, one person's needs might consistently be considered more important than the other's. And, of course, powerful, needy parents can continue to dominate the lives of their offspring until a ripe old age if the pattern remains unchallenged and unbroken.

When such a pattern is established early, it can be hard to break. If this pattern exists in your own life, you may choose your adult relationships based on finding someone to play this dominating role in your life, since this way of being has become what makes you feel comfortable—albeit one that undermines you. When you are dominated in this way, it becomes a great challenge to know yourself well and to identify your needs—and this is where problems start.

Extensions of this phenomenon can be found at many different levels in society. For example, we Westerners are all dominated by the high-tech, advertising-led modern world, which itself is dominated by materialistic values. We are dominated by left-brain, achievement-orientated education systems. We are dominated by reductionistic medicine. Those of a gentler, more spiritual nature often find themselves somewhat overwhelmed by these societal pressures. It is difficult for them to assert their own values and to create a lifestyle true to themselves, and this may lead to chronic compromise at many levels of life.

If people are very sensitive, the atmosphere or energy of a building or the geographical area in which they live may dominate them. Problems can also arise if people are forced to live in a country with a culture very different from their own, where the dominant values all around them are in conflict with their own underlying values or true nature.

Without realizing it, we may use a lot of energy to resist the dominant forces around us. The key here is to recognize the phenomenon in the first place. The minute you become aware that you are "under the power" of another person, value system, situation, or place, you can begin to do something about it.

The flip side of this dynamic is that those who allow themselves to be dominated can under other circumstances be very dominant. In the extreme, people who have been abused can themselves become abusers. To make this realization about oneself can be shattering, and it often requires a therapist's help to break the cycle. If you have been abused long term it may take a while to rebuild your sense of self once you are no longer being dominated. However, once embarked upon, the process of reclaiming your personal power will enrich and strengthen you and eventually give you an enormous sense of relief. In turn, your will and energy will rebound, and you will possess much stronger resources for your own healing and self-defense.

REORIENTING TO YOUR TRUE SELF

Almost inevitably, as you stop being the way other people want you to be, the question arises "Who is the real me?" You may never have had a chance to think about this question. People are constantly pressured by parents, teachers, and society to live up to their expectations, to be the way they want them to be, to follow their advice, or simply to "play the game."

Discovering Your Core Values

To find out for yourself what would be a fully authentic life, consider taking some quiet reflective time in a loving, supportive environment. This could be in retreat, in a therapeutic group, or with good friends who are aware you need time and space to reorient yourself. Start by doing a relaxation exercise, and then focus your attention on your heart area. Concentrate on generating loving feelings in the heart—either toward someone close to you or toward yourself, or a more generalized sense of compassion toward others. When you are in this loving "heart space," ask yourself:

- ❖ What is most important to me in life? What is it that really matters to me?

- ❖ In my heart of hearts, how do I want to spend the precious resources of my time and energy?

Write down your responses.

It is a good idea to repeat this exercise several times over several days. You will probably find that as the days pass you make a journey through deeper and deeper levels of yourself, until eventually you discover your innermost values. If this does not come easily to you, you could try imagining that you have been diagnosed with a terminal illness and have only a year to live. Then ask yourself what would be really important to you, and what you would want to do with your time and energy in your remaining year. Imagining this scenario has a tendency to sharpen the focus of the mind greatly.

Examining Your Will to Live

After looking more deeply within yourself, you may find that you are not really that excited to go on living at all. A big part of you may even long for death. Don't be afraid if you discover this. Freud asserted that all of us have equal and opposite urges—Thanatos, the urge toward death, and Eros, the urge toward life. Normally, people move back and forth between these poles, but some of us have a much stronger longing for death than others. Other people are so frightened of dying that an enormous amount of their energy is taken up trying to avoid even thinking about death, even if, underneath, they have lost the will to live.

To develop a deeper relationship with yourself, it can be very helpful to examine your feelings about death and dying to discover where your true motivation lies. It is said that people can only truly embrace life and live it to the fullest when they can also embrace the reality of death, and when the desire for death has been worked through to a point where they can genuinely make a choice for life.

Most people working in the holistic field view death not as failure or even necessarily as the end, but more as a transition. When you work in this profound territory, it is good to ask yourself if you really do have the will to live, or whether it has been beaten out of you by life's difficulties. If you feel ambivalent about life, deeply soul weary, or just plain lost, it may well be time to seek a combination of spiritual healing and transpersonal psychotherapy to help you rekindle your commitment to life and to find joy in living.

If you discover that your main purpose for living is your children or partner, then it may be worth exploring further to see whether there are unexpressed areas of yourself that need to emerge. These areas may have been abandoned as your life became focused on other things. While devotion to your nearest and dearest is absolutely right and wonderful, there's a better way to live than by living your life through others. Doing so can make you dependent on them and them on you, and in turn make it harder for them to have their own lives.

Living Life with Purpose and Meaning

Once you have a clear sense of what in life really matters to you and excites you, next you need to make sure that these priorities are reflected in the way you spend your time. If the best part of your life is squashed into a tiny fraction of your time, your soul or spirit will inevitably suffer. Once you know what your priorities are, try step by step to change the balance of time and energy in your life, and watch your health and happiness blossom as you become more and more alive.

Jung, one of the most significant psychologists of recent times, said that there is one state above all others that will surely kill a person—living life without meaning. For some, a sense of meaning comes from their inner life, their creativity, or their relationship to the divine. For others, it comes from a concrete focus, such as helping to house the homeless or feed the starving.

Increasingly, people are finding a personal meaning to life through their understanding and consciousness of the journey of their soul or spirit. People with a spiritual orientation often see themselves as spiritual beings in physical bodies. While anticipating their ultimate release at death back into the spiritual dimension, they seek to understand the purpose of their incarnation and to heed the lessons they are taught as they progress along life's path. This is consistent with the Eastern view of continuous reincarnation into different lifetimes until we learn enough not to need to come back anymore.

Whatever your belief, the important thing for the immune system is that you are as happy, excited, and committed to life as possible. Lawrence LeShan described this as "singing your own song"—feeling full of excitement when you wake up each day and full of gratitude as you go to sleep. For many people, such a state seems a long way from how they currently live. Our goal must be to seek this kind of happiness—breaking where necessary the addiction we have to suffering and the comfort of staying stuck in our safe but unsatisfying rut.

Self-Expression

Two of humans' great "soul" needs are the need for self-expression and the need to be recognized for who we are. We are each unique, and encouraging our personal forms of expression is fundamental for both individual health and the health of society. Unfortunately, the Puritan ethos and schooling most of us receive tends to encourage the reverse, squashing individuality and encouraging uniformity. Educational processes by and large tend to push children and students all through the same courses, so they achieve the same standards in the same subjects at the same age. In high school we are allowed to make some choices as we lean toward different career paths, but by this point the school system has lost the interest of a good percentage of children (in the UK, for instance, it is estimated that six out of seven young people lose interest in school by age fifteen). In fact, the way we are traditionally taught in schools takes advantage of only one of seven learning styles. Consequently, many children who go through the conventional school system will fail to fulfill their potential or to express themselves well in life.

It is vital for our health to redress the inhibiting influences in our educational system—and in all other areas of society as well. It is important at school, at home, at work, and in the community to enjoy the differences in people and to promote the unique skills they bring to situations. In particular, we must unlearn our prejudices and our practice of discriminating against people who choose an unconventional path. For yourself, be sure that the job you choose, the place where you live, the people with whom you have relationships, and your own sexuality, creativity, physicality, and appearance are all areas in which you can fully and truly express yourself.

If you dress to please others, stop immediately; dress in a way that pleases you. If you make love in a way you think is expected of you or that your partner likes, start discovering how you would like to express yourself sexually. If you live in a house that is full of your parents' old furniture, in an area you don't like, think about where and how you would like to live. If you have inherited a lot of your parents' things, you might find it amazingly refreshing to get rid of the history you are dragging around. Start defining your own taste; keep only one or two important possessions for their historic and sentimental value. If you are a physical person who loves to dance, run, or climb mountains, but have forgone these pursuits as you've grown older, get your body moving again. If your job isn't really you, find a way to change to one that more closely reflects your core values. You will be far more fulfilled.

If you feel limited or inhibited in your relationships, decide to change this pattern; learn to be exactly who you are. If you don't, others will suspect that you are not being yourself and will lose respect for you. There is nothing more off-putting than somebody who is inauthentic. If someone doesn't like or want to be with the real you, then it is time to leave the relationship anyway.

If you feel too vulnerable to let go of a "false" relationship, seek the support of a counselor to help you through the transition period. On the other hand, if you are dealing with problems in a long-term committed relationship, seeking counseling by yourself or jointly with your partner can help to change the relationship patterns.

If you believe you are too old to make these kinds of changes, let me reassure you it is never too late to "come home to yourself" and start leading an authentic life. I have witnessed hundreds of people of all ages who, when confronted with the diagnosis of cancer, made key changes in their lives. In the process, they came back to life in spirit, mind, and body.

SPIRITUAL NOURISHMENT

The next vital step is to find ways to nourish your spirit. Having read the last few pages, your spirit may already be jumping for joy at the thought of getting some recognition and attention, and being given permission to fully express yourself.

Many people grow up thinking spirituality equals religion, and they experience religion as something that represses rather than something that frees the spirit. Historically in the West, spirituality has been something that is acknowledged perhaps once a week on the traditional Sabbath, rather than something that is nurtured continuously. In the UK the Prince of Wales, in a millennium lecture, urged people to "rediscover or reacknowledge a sense of the sacred in our dealings with the natural world and with each other." By doing this we will *live* spirituality as opposed to keeping it in a separate compartment of our minds and lives.

Buddhists and yogis believe that the material world and even our emotions are illusions, and that the spiritual dimension is reality. They maintain that our preoccupation with the material world and with our sense of self prevents us from understanding the true nature of this reality and from experiencing the associated bliss and freedom.

Recognition of life's spiritual dimension is reaching unprecedented levels in our culture. People are consciously shifting their emphasis from material to spiritual values—often described as being "in transformation." When you meet people who no longer live in the grip of material values and the anxiety that goes with them, the difference is obvious. Invariably, these people say that the only thing to live for is the present moment, and that when you can do this with full loving attention, life becomes truly happy.

Mair Hoskins was diagnosed in 1998 with a very aggressive cancer that had already spread to her lymph nodes. She was offered radiation treatment and was advised by her consultant to "go home and live every day as if it were your last." She was shocked and put into deep despair by his words.

Her radiation involved staying at the oncology center in Bristol for five weeks. Mair had always had a gift for drawing but had failed to develop it. She had enrolled in a painting course earlier in the year but was too busy to follow it up. Now with so much time on her hands, waiting for appointments, she had the perfect opportunity to paint. She filled her time with painting and continued painting when she got home. At first it was just an experiment with pastels to occupy her time so she did not have to think about the cancer. But soon it became a great joy. She even sold two of her paintings to raise money to go to the Bristol Cancer Help Centre for a week with her husband. A year later, in November 2000, she wrote:

> The experience of Bristol was to change my life. As soon as I walked through the doors of the Centre I was greeted with such love and care from all the staff. There was nothing formal or intimidating about the Centre. There was a relaxed loving atmosphere that immediately put me at ease. Before, I had felt helpless about my situation, but gradually I began to feel more in control. There was something I could do for myself to improve my chances of survival. Changing my diet and eating healthy, healing foods was just the beginning. I became more aware of the whole of me—of my body, mind, and spirit, and getting them working together in harmony. Through meditation, relaxation, and visualization I began to find a peace within myself.

> On the Wednesday night of my week at Bristol, Pat Pilkington, one of the Centre's original founders, led us in a group-healing meditation. During the meditation I had a very special experience of God's love for me, and such an infilling of His Spirit that the joy I felt was inexpressible. It was an overwhelming and life-changing experience. And the joy is still with me over a year later. I can honestly say that the happiness I felt then I still feel now. I was brought out of a place of dark despair into the healing light of God's love. It has given me a burning desire to help and encourage others going through similar times of crisis and challenge.

> Before I had cancer, I was too busy to do the things I really wanted to do. I rushed about, not stopping long enough to appreciate the beauty around me, and was always looking forward to the next project. Now I am living my life moment by moment, savoring the little things that I once took for granted, experiencing all the wonderful things around me, and expressing my joy in the art form that I love.

> I have so much to be grateful for—all the staff at Bristol and their loving care and the strategies they gave me in my fight against cancer, the love and support of a wonderful husband, my

children, all my family and friends, the prayers of a supportive Church—and, most of all, the assurance of God's love for me, which I received that night at the Bristol Cancer Help Centre.

I have witnessed this transformational process over and over again at the Bristol Cancer Help Centre, as the shock of a cancer diagnosis awakens people to the reality of their spiritual nature. For others, fleeting glimpses of their spiritual nature and connection to life may come at moments of intense joy, pain, or beauty, through sexual union with another, while meditating, or through experiencing true communion with God or the Holy Spirit. Sometimes people reach this state under the influence of consciousness-raising drugs. What is important is recognizing that each of us has our own way of experiencing the spiritual dimension, and finding our own way to do this.

As we explore our spiritual life may confront a paradox: On the one hand, we must make the effort to find our individuality and to express our true nature, while, on the other hand, we must learn to "let go and let God." The challenge is to live fully in the world while retaining a sense of a greater spiritual reality and our ability to let go into a bigger Truth—to be "in the world but not of it."

The appreciation of these different levels of reality comes from a shift in our perception or consciousness. In everyday consciousness, we need our ego, a strong sense of self, and the will to live our unique purpose. But from time to time we get above the clouds, so to speak, and see the greater reality, appreciating the tiny part we play in the vast process of life. From this perspective, the daily pressures and priorities of our existence seem quite unimportant. Once you experience this other perspective, you will not let your life be as driven or stressed, or get as lost in your "personal drama," and will perhaps even stop taking yourself quite so seriously!

When developing individual spirituality, it is important to be completely authentic. People can spend years going to church or sitting in meditation groups following other people's recipes for the spiritual life, feeling absolutely nothing at all. If you are doing this,

I suggest you stop right away and do something more profitable with your time.

As I watch people unfold into their own sense of spirit and spirituality, I notice recurring themes. One universal source of spiritual uplift is beauty, and those who embrace their spirituality consistently aim to bring more and more beauty into life, whether this be through nature, the home, clothes, art, or exquisite music. In Japan, there is a group called the Johrei Society whose fundamental philosophy maintains that health depends on three things: respect for the environment and eating organic food; daily spiritual healing within the family context; and the central place of beauty in life. Before coming across this group, I had never seen the need for beauty expressed so strongly, but the more I think about it, the more I agree that beauty in our lives is central to our spiritual health. If people live in an ugly concrete jungle, they can become starved of the uplift offered by natural beauty. Making time to catch the dawn or climbing to the top of a mountain to see for miles around can be greatly uplifting to the spirit.

Another key to spiritual nourishment is simply taking time and space for yourself, as I mention over and over in this book. Often, the spirit longs for simplicity, for time to "be" rather than "do." If you find it impossible to rest or have space in your own home, it may be worth going on retreat. A growing number of centers offer the opportunity to have time to oneself in a supportive, loving atmosphere, either with or without spiritual guidance. Taking regular time to come home to yourself and to deepen your sense of spiritual connection in this way is profoundly healing and nurturing and is the best possible form of preventive medicine you can give yourself. If you already have a strong sense of spirit or embrace a particular religious faith, you may wish to seek a retreat center that supports your beliefs. But there are plenty of nonsectarian retreat centers for those who wish to explore their spirituality in a less structured environment (see the Resources section). Many retreat centers allow people to study or deepen meditation techniques. Doing this in a dedicated way with the support of others can make it easier to maintain the practice at home.

The most fundamental spiritual value of all is the need to give and receive love—in our personal relationships and in our relationship to God or Spirit. For some, their spiritual problem is that they have a great deal of love to give but no way to express it, while others feel desperately in need of love and attention. If your ability to give and receive love feels blocked, or you are deprived of love because of social circumstances, it is a very good idea, either through therapeutic relationships, support groups, or spiritual healing, to find ways to give and receive love in a safe context.

Many groups and workshops embrace a strongly supportive, loving ethos. It is amazing how people who attend these workshops can receive high-quality love and support from people who were total strangers only a few days earlier. We tend to get stuck in the idea that, to be meaningful, love must come from a partner, close friends, or family. Fortunately, more and more ways to develop trust and meaningful connection with others are available that invite us to develop and enjoy a more open sense of being part of a universal family. Positive feelings are generated in yoga groups, meditation classes, support groups, tantric yoga groups, and a host of other growth and developmental workshops (see the Resources section). As with finding the right therapist, it is always wise to evaluate group facilitators for their skill, experience, warmth, and professionalism, taking note of their reputation before signing up.

For many people, an important outlet for love and caring is volunteer work. If, for example, you feel frustrated because all your children have left home and you are without a partner, it may be deeply satisfying to work with those in need within your community. However, try to balance the love you give others with the love you give yourself and receive from others.

A completely different way of generating and expressing love is through a form of Buddhist meditation called *metta bharvana* (pronounced *parvana*). *Metta bharvana* involves sitting in meditation and gradually focusing attention on the heart area. First, you generate loving feelings toward someone you find easy to love, like a child, parent, or partner. Then, gradually visualize extending your love to a wider circle of family and friends. Next, you extend the loving feeling to your colleagues and acquaintances; then extend this feeling to the whole community or town in which you live, to your state, country, and so on. If you feel able to, extend this feeling of compassion around the world, until you are literally holding the world in your heart. As you become more comfortable with this practice, you can specifically include people you dislike or have disagreements with, holding them in your heart until you can genuinely extend love toward them. The process also provides an ideal opportunity to include yourself as a recipient of your own love. Similar benefits occur as a result of prayer or during absent healing.

Developing a sense of compassion for yourself and others makes the process of forgiveness and living in harmony much easier. When you work on the inner plane, you rapidly change the template or program with which you live the whole of your life. Once you hold your enemies in compassion, your relationships with them will very quickly change. Likewise, holding yourself in compassion is the quickest way to develop a better relationship with yourself. Such an attitude shift will make adopting all the other health-promoting changes suggested in this book far, far easier.

6

❖

Getting Started

Having read this far you may feel daunted or overwhelmed by the number of things you need to think about and do in order to reduce your risk of cancer. However, for most of us the most important areas to address include eating healthy food, giving up smoking, drinking in moderation, getting regular exercise, and reducing stress. This may still sound like an awful lot, and ultimately you may need to address all of these issues, but try to start with the one you think is the most significant offender in your case. Establish a clear intention to change, and arrange for all the support you need to succeed in making the change. As you progress, tackle the next priority issue, continuing step by step until you are in good health. Remember what has been emphasized throughout the book: If you are low in energy and/or emotionally vulnerable, you need emotional support to change—maybe in the form of counseling, spiritual healing, or energy medicines—before beginning self-help activities.

Finally, it is very important to avoid feeling paranoid about getting cancer; our state of mind greatly affects the state of our immune system and overall health. You will not help yourself by getting into a state of anxious preoccupation about the matter. Instead, make the process of reducing your cancer risk as enjoyable as possible, involving friends, colleagues, and members of your family.

If you lose your way, be easy on yourself; pick up the book again and see what steps you can take to gently get yourself back on track. If you feel defeated, it may be time to seek the help of a holistic doctor to guide and support you through the process. Many holistic doctors, such as myself, who specialize in the holistic treatment of cancer, are more than delighted to provide the necessary support, encouragement, and guidance for anyone who wishes to reduce their cancer risk. Once you are healthier and happier, enjoying a strong immune system and good diet, you will be at lower risk from environmental hazards. But continue to take good care of yourself—protect yourself in the sun and around chemicals, medicines, and electromagnetic radiation, and practice safe sex.

Once you get your individual act together, it is time to get active socially and environmentally. All of us who are concerned about cancer prevention must lobby vociferously for the adoption of anticancer policies in all areas of life. A good place to start is by making sure our children and the generations that follow can eat balanced healthy diets, get safe nutritious food, and live in a smoke- and pollution-free environment. We must also act to clean up our environment and work hard to restore this extraordinary planet to its exquisitely beautiful natural state.

We cannot wait for our governments to act. We must make thinking about and eradicating cancer an urgent personal priority. In tackling this issue we will also be confronting many of the other problems that wreck lives and cause immeasurable human suffering.

Please wake up now to the urgent need to take action. Commit yourself today to getting involved in cancer prevention, first in your own life and then as part of a wider movement, so that our grandchildren may look back on cancer as a nasty moment in history. Never has there been a clearer indication that we have drifted off course than the fact that the cells of our bodies are mutating and growing out of control. Never has there been a greater imperative to act to restore health and balance to ourselves and to our beautiful but endangered planet.

Appendix 1

Chemicals in the Environment Known to Disrupt the Endocrine System

- Cadmium
- DDT and its degradation products
- Di-(2)-ethyl hexphtalate (DEHP)
- Dicofol
- EBDC fungicides
- Hexachlorobenzene (HCB)
- Kelthane
- Kepone
- Lead
- Lindane and other hexachlorocyclohexane congeners
- Mercury
- Methoxychlor
- Octachloro styrene
- PCB congeners (some)
- Synthetic pyrethroids

- ❖ Triazine herbicides
- ❖ 2, 3, 7, 8-TCDD and other dioxins
- ❖ 2, 3, 7, 8-TCDDF and other furans
- ❖ Tributyltin and other organotin compounds
- ❖ Alkyl phenols (non-biodegradable detergents and antioxidants present in modified polystyrene and PVCs)
- ❖ Styrene dimers and trimers

Appendix 2

Chemicals Found in Household Products and Their Effects

Chemicals contained in household products that are either carcinogenic (affecting the cells of the body) or teratogenic (affecting the germ cells, i.e., the cells of the sperm and ovaries):

Chemical	Effect	Found in
Acetoxyphenylmercury	Teratogenic	Paints
Acid blue 9	Carcinogenic	Toilet-bowl cleaners and deodorizers
Aluminum silicate	Some evidence of carcinogenicity in the dry state	Some paints
Artificial coal tar colors that contain lead and arsenic	Carcinogenic	Black and brown hair dyes
Benzene	Carcinogenic	Some adhesives
Bronopol	Breaks down to formaldehyde, which is carcinogenic	Cosmetics
Cadmium	Carcinogenic and teratogenic	Some oil paints

Chemical	Effect	Found in
Cobalt	Carcinogenic	Some oil paints
Crystalline silica	Carcinogenic in the dry state	Cleansers, cat litter, powdered flea-control products
1, 4-dichlorobenzene (para-dichlorobenzene)	Carcinogenic	Moth repellents, toilet deodorizers
Dichlorvos (DDVP)	Carcinogenic, teratogenic	Some no-pest strips, flea collars, and pet-flea-control products
Diethanolamine (DEA)	Reacts with nitrites to form nitrosamines, which are carcinogenic	Wide range of household cleaning products, cosmetics
Dioctyl phthalate	Carcinogenic	Adhesives and correction fluid
Ethoxylated alcohols	May be contaminated with 1, 4-dioctane, which is carcinogenic	Cosmetics
Formaldehyde	Carcinogenic	Some furniture polishes, cleaners, waxes, and a wide range of consumer items, especially paints and related products
Hexachlorobenzene (HCB)	Carcinogenic	Some oil paints
Hydramethylnon	Carcinogenic	Some household and garden pesticides
Lanolin (not toxic on its own, but may be contaminated with DDT, dieldrin, lindane, diazinon, and other pesticides)	Carcinogenic	Cosmetics and body and hand creams
Lead	Carcinogenic	Some oil paints
Medium aliphatic-	Some evidence	Some car waxes

Chemical	Effect	Found in
hydrocarbons	suggesting carcinogenicity	
Methoxychlor	Limited evidence of carcinogenicity	Some pet-flea-control products
Methyl chloride (dichloromethane)	Carcinogenic	Some paint strippers and spray paints
Morpholine	Reacts with nitrites to form carcinogenic nitrosamines	Some furniture polishes
Naled	Transformation products include dichlorvos, which is carcinogenic	Some pet-flea-control products
Ortho phenylphenols	Probably carcinogenic	Some air fresheners and disinfectants
Padimate-O	Can cause the formation of nitrosamines, which arecarcinogenic	Sun screens and cosmetics
Permethrin	Carcinogenic	Some household and garden pesticides and pet-flea-control products
Petroleum distillates, hydrocarbons, process oils, solvents, and spirits	May contain traces of benzene, which is carcinogenic	Some furniture polishes
Polychlorinated biphenyls (PCBs)	Carcinogenic and teratogenic	Some oil paints
Propylene oxide	Carcinogenic	Some adhesives
Rotenone	Carcinogenic	Some pet-flea-control products

Chemical	Effect	Found in
Sodium 2,4-dichloro-phenoxyacetate	Carcinogenic	Herbicides in lawn-care products
Sodium ortho-phenylphenol	Carcinogenic	Some bathroom cleaners
Solvent orange 3 dye; solvent red 4 dye; blue 1; green 3; D and C red 33; F, D, and C yellow 5; F, D, and C yellow 6	Carcinogenic	Some polishes, cosmetics
Talc	Carcinogenic when inhaled	Cosmetics and some household and garden pesticides
Tetrachloroethylene (perchlorethylene)	Carcinogenic	Some spot removers
Tetrachlorvinphos	Carcinogenic	Some pet-flea-control products
Titanium dioxide	Limited evidence of carcinogenicity	Some paints and shoe polishes
Triethanolamine (TEA)	Can react with nitrites to form carcinogenic nitrosamines	Some liquid all-purpose cleaning products, metal polishes, spot removers, and other household cleaning products, and cosmetics
Trisodium nitrylotriacetate	Carcinogenic	Some bathroom cleaning products

Appendix 3

Occupational Cancer-Risk Factors

Susceptible Workers	Likely Carcinogenic Agent	Risk
Asbestos workers, miners, shipyard workers, insulators, rubber-tire-plant workers, demolition workers, brake liners	Asbestos fibers	Mesothelioma, cancer of the lung and pharynx (throat)
Brick and ceramic manufacturers/workers	Arsenic, beryllium, and chromium	Cancer of the skin, lung, nose, throat, and liver
Cadmium production workers, metal workers, electroplaters	Cadmium	Cancer of the lung and prostate
Chemical industry workers	Amino-biphenyl	Leukemia
	Benzene	Cancer of the pancreas
	Benzidine	Cancer of the bladder
	Chloromethyl ether	Cancer of the lung
	Cadmium	Cancer of the prostate
	Chromium, 2-naphthylamine	Cancer of the throat
Chromium and alloy production workers	Chromium and chromium compounds	Cancer of the lung, nose, and pharynx (throat)
Chromium and alloy production workers	Chromium and chromium compounds	Cancer of the lung, nose, and pharynx (throat)

Susceptible Workers	Likely Carcinogenic Agent	Risk
Coal, gas, and shale-oil production workers	Aromatic hydrocarbons	Cancer of the lung, skin, bladder, and pancreas
Coke plant workers	Coke-oven gases and vapors	Cancer of the lung, skin, bladder, and pancreas
Copper production smelters, electrolyzers	2-naphthylamine	Cancer of the bladder and pancreas
Dye-industry workers	Aminebiphenyl, benzidine, and 2-naphthylamine	Cancer of the bladder and pancreas
Electrical/electronic workers, electricians, radio/TV repairers, telephone and computer mechanics	Electromagnetic fields (EMF), beryllium	Leukemia, lymphomas, cancer of the brain and bladder
Electroplaters/electrolyzers	Cadmium and 2-naphthylamine	Cancer of the prostate, bladder, and pancreas
Farmers and agricultural workers	Ultraviolet radiation, pesticides, weed killers	Leukemia, lymphoma, soft-tissue sarcoma, cancer of the skin, lip, prostate, and lung
Garage and transport workers	Diesel exhaust	Cancer of the lung
Glass manufacture workers	Arsenic, chromium compounds	Cancer of the skin, lung, liver, nose, and throat
Hairdressers	Hair dyes	Cancer of the bladder
Insulators	Asbestos fibers	Mesothelioma, cancer of the lung and pharynx (throat)
Leather- and shoe-industry workers	Benzene, isopropyl	Leukemia, cancer of the sinuses
Nickel production workers	Nickel 2-naphthylamine	Cancer of the nose, bladder, and pancreas

Susceptible Workers	Likely Carcinogenic Agent	Risk
Nuclear power workers	Beryllium cadmium	Cancer of the bladder, lung, and prostate
Office workers	Tobacco smoke	Cancer of the lung and throat
Painters	Painting materials, benzene	Leukemia, cancer of the lung
Petroleum workers	Arsenic, benzene, and petroleum	Leukemia, cancer of the skin, lung, gallbladder, and bile duct
Plastics industry workers	Vinyl chloride	Lymphomas, cancer of the liver and lung
Radiologists, radiographers, nurses	Ionizing radiation, cancer drugs	Leukemia, myeloma, cancer of the skin, thyroid, brain, lung, breast, bone, and pancreas
Rubber-tire-manufacture workers	Asbestos fibers, benzene, auramine, and 2-naphthylamine	Mesothelioma, leukemia, cancer of the lung, bladder, pancreas, gallbladder, and bile duct
Steelworkers	Coke-oven gases and vapors	Cancer of the lung and kidney
Tanners	Arsenic	Cancer of the skin and lung
Uranium miners	Ionizing radiation and radon gas	Leukemia, myeloma, cancer of the skin, thyroid, brain, lung, breast, bone, and pancreas
Waiters/bartenders	Tobacco smoke	Cancer of the lung and pharynx (throat)
Woodworkers, carpenters, furniture makers, polishers and finishers	Wood dust and benzene	Leukemia, cancer of the nose, sinuses, and pharynx (throat)

Appendix 4

Risk Factors for Specific Cancers

Anal Cancer

❖ genetic inheritance

❖ infection with certain types of the sexually transmitted infection human papillomavirus (HPV), most frequently types 16 and 18

❖ anal fissures and fistulas

❖ anal intercourse

❖ immunosuppressive drugs

❖ smoking (possibly)

Bladder Cancer

❖ smoking

❖ painkillers containing phenacetin (now withdrawn from sale)

❖ bladder papilloma

❖ artificial sweeteners (possibly)

❖ high coffee consumption

❖ recurrent bladder infections

❖ radiation to the pelvis

❖ occupational exposure to aromatic amines, paints, hairdressing products, printing products

Cancer of the Bowel

❖ genetic inheritance (15 percent of cases are inherited)

❖ a high-calorie diet with excess fat, sugar, meat (especially red), and salt

❖ a diet low in vegetables, fruit, fiber, fish, and calcium

❖ being overweight

❖ physical inactivity

❖ high alcohol consumption (more than three units a day for men and two units a day for women) over a period of twenty years

❖ smoking (thought to account for 10 percent of bowel cancers)

Brain Tumors

❖ genetic inheritance (in association with neurofibromatosis)

❖ use of pesticides and insecticides

❖ exposure to petrochemicals, rubber, and vinyl chloride; electromagnetic fields (in electrical and electronic-industry workers); radiation (in radiologists and radiographers); and uranium (in uranium miners)

❖ head injuries (slightly increased risk of meningioma)

❖ excessive number of dental X rays (slightly increased risk of meningioma and glioma)

❖ nitrate-containing foods, e.g., sausages and salamis

❖ smoking (possibly)

❖ exposure to low-frequency electromagnetic fields from living or playing near high-tension electricity wires (possible risk for children)

Breast Cancer

❖ genetic inheritance

❖ alcohol (more than 2 units a day)

❖ high hormone levels due to obesity, diet, HRT, or the Pill (and, possibly, environmental estrogen-mimicking substances called xenoestrogens)

❖ physical inactivity

❖ excessive radiation of the chest

❖ a high-calorie diet with excess meat and fat

❖ obesity

❖ low vegetable and fiber intake

Cervical Cancer

❖ infection with certain types of the human papillomavirus (HPV), most frequently types 16 and 18

❖ abnormalities in the mucus membrane of the cervix (CIN 1, 2, and 3)

❖ abnormalities in the mucus membrane of the vagina or skin of the vulva

❖ unsafe sex

❖ smoking

❖ a diet low in vegetables, fruit, beta-carotene, vitamin C, and folic acid

Cancer of the Esophagus (Gullet)

❖ genetic inheritance

❖ Barrett's esophagus, a condition in which there is reflux of the contents of the stomach into the esophagus, which over time causes inflammation, scarring, narrowing, or out-pouching

❖ alcohol

❖ smoking

❖ smoked, pickled, cured, and preserved foods

❖ low intake of beta-carotene and vitamins C and E

Gallbladder Cancer

❖ genetic inheritance where there is a tendency toward cholesterol gallstones (gallstones are more common with multiple pregnancies, obesity, a high-calorie diet, and a diet low in fruit, vegetables, and grains)

❖ gallstones, especially if they are big and the gallbladder wall is calcified

❖ occupational exposure to products used in the car-manufacturing, petroleum, rubber, and textile industries

Kidney Cancer

❖ genetic inheritance in association with nonpolyposis colorectal cancer syndrome

❖ occupational exposure to leather dyes, textile dyes, rubber, plastic, coke ovens, cadmium, asbestos, petroleum, tar, and pitch products

❖ phenacetin painkillers (now withdrawn from sale)

❖ some diuretics and antihypertensive drugs and diet pills

❖ kidney injury

❖ radiation

❖ long-term hemodialysis

❖ large kidney stones

❖ smoking

❖ being overweight

Leukemias

❖ genetic inheritance (very rarely, but higher risk in those with Down's syndrome)

❖ occupational exposure to products used in the chemical industry, shoe trade, and uranium mining; exposure to the solvent benzene (also found in unleaded fuel), radiation, and low-frequency electromagnetic fields (in electrical and electronic-industry workers), and pesticides (in farmers)

❖ previous radiation exposure from diagnostic X rays or radiotherapy

❖ chemotherapy with melphalan and chlorambucil

❖ the antibiotics chloramphenicol and phenylbutazone

❖ smoking (possibly)

Liver Cancer

❖ alcohol (intake of more than two to three units a day)

❖ smoking (possibly)

❖ genetic inheritance (very rarely)

❖ past hepatitis B and hepatitis C infection

❖ exposure to aflatoxin in tropical countries (especially Africa)

❖ chronic liver disease, e.g., liver cirrhosis

❖ previous steroid use, especially androgenic anabolic steroids

❖ oral contraceptives (possibly)

❖ previous blood transfusion

Lung Cancer

❖ smoking, which causes 85 percent of lung cancers. About one in five people now living in developed countries will be killed by tobacco unless smoking habits change. This amounts to 250 million people, or the entire population of the United States. Most alarming is the increase in female deaths from smoking. Lung cancer has overtaken breast cancer as the major cause of death among women in Scotland and northern England, and that may soon be the case in the entire UK. In Britain, smoking causes 100,000 deaths every year, 50,000 of which are due to cancer. This is the same as a jumbo jet crashing every day and killing all of the passengers on board. Sound incredibly high? Compare this to U.S. figures, where it is estimated that over 430,000 people die every year from diseases directly related to smoking.

❖ radon gas. Based on a national residential radon survey completed in 1991, the average indoor radon level in the United States is 1.3 picocuries per liter (pCi/L). The average outdoor level is about 0.4 pCi/L. The EPA considers 4 pCi/L as its "action" level. In the United States, about 10 percent of deaths from lung cancer are believed to be attributable to radon—only smoking causes more deaths from lung cancer.

❖ chronic lung disease

❖ excessive radiation to the chest

❖ secondhand smoke

❖ asbestos

❖ occupational exposure to nickel and chromium compounds and arsenic

❖ occupational exposure to asbestos (especially in those who smoke)

❖ a diet low in vegetables

❖ a diet high in meat and fat

Lymphomas

Hodgkin's Lymphoma

❖ genetic inheritance

❖ occupational exposure to tar and benzene (in woodworkers, rubber workers, and chemical workers)

❖ tonsil removal

❖ amphetamine usage

❖ use of the drug phenytoin in epilepsy (possibly)

❖ viral infection in glandular fever with Epstein-Barr

❖ immune deficiency

Non-Hodgkin's Lymphoma

❖ genetic inheritance

❖ occupational exposure to chlorophenols, phenoxy acids, asbestos, benzene, radiation, uranium, low-frequency electromagnetic fields, pesticides, herbicides, and fertilizers

❖ viral infection with Epstein-Barr viruses and viruses associated with AIDS

❖ poor and suppressed immunity

❖ immunosuppressive drugs, especially after a kidney transplant

❖ use of the drug phenytoin for epilepsy

❖ radiation treatment

Melanoma

❖ excessive sunlight (90 percent of cases)

❖ genetic inheritance (2 percent of cases)

❖ compromised immune function (with coexisting leukemia or lymphoma, or when using immunosuppressive drugs, e.g., after transplants)

❖ radiation

❖ multiple skin moles

❖ use of tanning beds

❖ chronic leg ulcers

❖ occupational exposure to tar, asphalt, pitch, waxes, heavy oils (including shale oil), and arsenic

❖ a diet low in vitamin A, beta-carotene, and vitamin C

❖ high fat intake

Mouth and Throat Cancer

❖ occupational exposure to nickel and asbestos, and mustard gas (historically)

❖ sunlight (especially for cancer of the lip)

❖ leukoplakia

❖ radiation

❖ infection with Epstein-Barr virus

❖ use of tobacco, snuff, or marijuana

❖ alcohol

❖ repeated irritation or abrasions in the mouth

❖ a diet low in vitamins C, E, and beta-carotene

Cancer of the Pancreas

❖ genetic inheritance

❖ occupational exposure to nickel, copper, and asbestos (in chemical and dye workers), uranium (in rubber workers), and radiation (in radiologists and radiographers)

❖ chronic pancreatitis (inflammation of the pancreas)

❖ diabetes (slightly increases risk)

❖ smoking

❖ a diet high in fat and meat with low vegetable and fruit intake

❖ high alcohol consumption

Cancer of the Penis

❖ infection with certain types of the sexually transmitted infection human papillomavirus (HPV), most frequently types 16 and 18

❖ in the uncircumcised, a narrowed foreskin coupled with poor hygiene

❖ unsafe anal sex, risking infection of the above viruses

❖ occupational exposure (in farmers) to fertilizers, pesticides, and weed killers

❖ smoking

Prostate Cancer

Possible risk factors (the causes of prostate cancer are still not well understood):

❖ high testosterone levels or high testosterone/estrogen ratios

❖ a high-fat diet

❖ genetic inheritance

❖ physical inactivity

❖ smoking (which increases the testosterone/estrogen ratio)

❖ occupational exposure to pesticides (in farmers) and cadmium (in battery and alloy workers and during electroplating)

❖ obesity

❖ a diet low in beta-carotene and foods containing vitamin E

❖ low intake of green leafy vegetables

❖ inadequate sunlight with resulting low levels of vitamin D

❖ vasectomy at a young age

❖ smoking

Sarcomas
(Cancers of the Bones or Connective Tissues)

❖ genetic inheritance in association with von Recklinghausen's disease (rarely)

❖ occupational exposure to herbicides, wood preservatives, radiation, and defoliants

❖ Paget's disease of the bone (where cartilage grows into the bone)

❖ radiation and chemotherapy treatments

❖ HIV infection progressing to AIDS—Kaposi's sarcoma

❖ metallic surgical implants

❖ bullet and shrapnel fragments in the body's connective tissue

❖ smoking

Stomach Cancer

❖ family history

❖ type A blood group (increases the risk by 20 percent)

❖ infection with the bacterium Helicobacter pylori

❖ previous surgical removal of part of the stomach (can have an effect fifteen to forty years later)

❖ pernicious anemia where there is no normal stomach-acid production

❖ all conditions that cause low stomach acid

❖ a diet low in vegetables, fruit, cereals, beta-carotene, and vitamins C and E

❖ a diet high in pickled, salted, or cured foods, or foods preserved in nitrate such as salami, sausages, hot dogs, smoked meat, smoked fish, or pickled food (all of which cause production of carcinogenic nitrosamines in the bowel)

❖ smoking

Testicular Cancer

❖ genetic inheritance (very rarely)

❖ occupational exposure to defoliants (in Vietnam veterans)

❖ undescended testicles

❖ mumps orchitis (inflammation of the testicles due to mumps)

❖ maternal use of diethylstilbestrol (otherwise known as DES and banned since 1965)

❖ synthetic estrogens in food

❖ a sedentary lifestyle

❖ tight pants

Thyroid Cancer

❖ genetic inheritance

❖ occupational exposure to ionizing radiation (in radiologists, radiographers, and uranium miners)

❖ excessive alcohol consumption

❖ preexisting thyroid illness

❖ exposure to radiation (since 1987, more than one thousand children in the Chernobyl area have developed cancer of the thyroid due to exposure to radioactive iodine after the nuclear accident)

Cancer of the Uterus and Ovaries

❖ genetic inheritance—in association with hereditary nonpolyposis colorectal cancer or breast/ovarian cancer syndrome

❖ previous breast, colorectal, ovarian, or uterine cancer

❖ use of estrogen-only HRT (increases the risk of uterine cancer more than ovarian cancer)

❖ polycystic ovaries

❖ use of fertility drugs (raises ovarian cancer risk)

❖ tamoxifen, the estrogen-blocking drug used to help prevent breast cancer or its recurrence (increases risk to the endometrium or lining of the uterus)

❖ long menstrual life with periods starting before age twelve and finishing after fifty years of age

❖ not having children

- high blood pressure or diabetes
- a high-calorie and high-fat diet
- a diet low in vegetables, fruit, and fish
- being overweight
- physical inactivity
- never having used the birth control pill

Vaginal and Vulval Cancer

- maternal use of diethylstilbestrol (otherwise known as DES and banned since 1965)
- infection with certain types of the human papillomavirus (HPV), most frequently types 16 and 18
- abnormalities in the skin or mucus membrane of the vulva or vagina
- radiation treatment
- extensive sexual activity in the very young, without adequate protection (high risk of sexually transmitted diseases)
- smoking

Appendix 5

Anticancer Foods and the Phytochemicals They Contain

Food	Phytochemicals
Alfalfa	Saponins, sterols, flavonoids, coumarins and alkaloids, vitamins and minerals
Alliums: onions, spring onions, garlic, leeks, chives	Allium compounds diallyl sulfide and allyl methyl trisulfide
Almonds	Protease inhibitors, phytate, genistein, lignins, and benzaldehyde
Apples	Chlorogenic acid and caffeic acid
Brassicas: broccoli, cabbage, brussels sprouts, collards, kale, bok choy, kohlrabi, arugula, horseradish, radish, rutabagas, and turnips	Dithiolthiones, isothyocyanates, glucosinolates, indole-3-carbinol, and sulfurophane (in broccoli)
Sprouted broccoli and cauliflower seeds	Sulfurophane (10–100 times higher levels than in the vegetables themselves)
Burdock root (gobo)—a component of the cancer remedy essiac	Benzaldehyde, phytosterols, glycosides, mokko lactone, and arctic acid
Citrus fruits	Coumarins and D-limonene, hesperatin, narangenin, glutathione, and bioflavonoids

Food	Phytochemicals
Flaxseed oil	Omega-3 essential fatty acids and antioxidants
Garlic	Selenium, germanium, antioxidants, isoflavones, and allyl sulfide
Ginger	Antioxidants, gingerol, and carotenes
Grapes	Antioxidants and ellagic acid (raisins also contain tannins and caffeic acid)
Licorice	Triterpenoids
Linseeds	Lignins and omega-3 essential fatty acids and alpha linolenic acid
Mushrooms (maitake, rei-shi, shiitake)	Polysaccharide immune stimulants (which boost interferon and interleukin levels), selenium, antioxidants, lignins, and adaptogenic compounds
Nettles	Carotenes, chlorophyll, folic acid, and selenium
Fresh nuts and seeds, particularly almonds, walnuts, black walnuts, pecans, sunflower seeds, sesame seeds, and linseeds (flaxseeds)	Protease inhibitors, essential fats, and antioxidants
Olive oil	Specific antioxidants
Orange/red/purple-colored foods such as apricots, cantaloupe, carrots, yellow and red peppers, beets, squashes, sweet potatoes, red and black berries	Beta-carotene and proanthocyanadins (among the most powerful antioxidants known)
Parsley	Phytosterols, carotenes, folic acid, chlorophyll, vitamin C, the essential oils terpenes and pinenes, and polyacetylene
Pineapple	Bromelain; protease inhibitors; citric, folic, malic and chlorogenic acids

Food	Phytochemicals
Potatoes	Protease inhibitors, chlorogenic acid, and vitamin C
Legumes and beans	Protease inhibitors, lignins, genistein, and phytosetrols
Brown rice	Rice bran saccharide
Seaweeds (kombu, kelp, nori, arame, laver bread, dulse, wakame)	Antioxidants, carotenes, selenium, iodine, alginic acid, the full range of minerals and trace elements, and vitamin B12
Soy products	The isoflavones genistein and diadzein, phytic acid, saponins, phytosterols, protease inhibitors, omega-3 fatty acids, and lecithin
Teas:	
Black tea	The polyphenols theaflavin and thearubigin (which interfere with the initiation, promotion, and growth stages of cancer)
Green tea	Epicatechin (the strongest antimutagen of any plant yet examined) and epigallocatechin-3-gallate
All leaf teas	Antimutagenic tannins, antioxidants, and polyphenols
Tomatoes	Antioxidants, flavonoids, lycopene, chlorogenic acid, coumarins, carotenes, and carotenoids
Turmeric	Curcumin

For a full explanation of the scientifically researched properties of these phytochemicals, see Suzannah Olivier's book *The Breast Cancer Prevention and Recovery Diet.*

Glossary

Adducts—chemical additions to DNA that distort its structure

Adenomatous—relating to an adenoma, an outgrowth of the mucus-membrane lining of the bowel

Aflatoxin—a metabolic product of a fungus that contaminates grains stored in hot and humid conditions

Aneuploidy—loss or gain of a single chromosome

Apoptosis—cell death

Beta-agonists—substances that stimulate beta-adrenaline receptors in the body

Carcinogenesis—the process by which cancer develops

Carcinogens—cancer-causing agents

Catechins—anticancer substance found in green tea

Cell lineage—the generations of cells descended from a parent cell

DNA—deoxyribonucleic acid, the main constituent of the chromosomes of all organisms

Endocrine system—the body's hormonal system

Free radicals—chemically active compounds that can cause DNA damage

Genome—the complement of single chromosomes contained in a nucleus, i.e., half of the twenty-three pairs of chromosomes

Leukemia—disease in which white blood cells are overproduced by bone marrow– and blood-forming organs

Lymphoma—a malignant tumor of the lymph nodes

Melanoma—a malignant tumor of the melanin-forming cells (usually in the skin)

Mesothelioma—cancer of the lining of the lung

Metastases—secondary cancers in tissues or organs distant from the site of origin of a cancer

Mind/body techniques—techniques (such as meditation, relaxation, and visualization) that affect the state of mind and subsequently the state of the body

Mutagens—substances that induce genetic changes that may lead to cancer

Mutations—changes in DNA, the genetic material of all living organisms

Myeloma—disease of the bone marrow

Neurotoxicity—toxicity to nerve tissue

Nitrosamines—carcinogenic compounds formed from nitrites or nitrates

Oncogenes—cancer genes

Pharmacogenetic polymorphisms—genetic susceptibility to environmental chemicals

Phytochemicals—plant chemicals that protect against cancer

Polycyclic aromatic hydrocarbons—cancer-causing chemicals found in smoke

Protease inhibitors—substances that inhibit the protein-digesting enzymes thought to protect cells from ionizing radioactivity

Proto-oncogenes—genes that normally control cell growth and proliferation but which can become mutated in one or two steps, facilitating the development of a cancer

Psychoneuroimmunology (PNI)—the study of how the mind and body are linked

Sarcoma—cancer of the bones or connective tissues

Teratogenic—producing cancerous change in the sperm or egg tissues, which can then be passed to offspring

Toxins—cell poisons

Resources

Holistic Doctors

Dr. Michael Lerner
Commonweal
PO Box 316
Bolinas CA 94924   (415) 868-0970
Website: www.commonweal.org

Dr. Rosy Daniel
General Inquiries:
Health Creation
77a, Alma Rd.
Bristol BS6 5HR, U.K.
Consultations:
The Harley Street Clinic — Oncology Unit
81 Harley St.
London W1N 1DE, UK   +44-20-7299-9428
(cancer patient inquiries only)

Dr. O. Carl Simonton, M.D.
Simonton Cancer Center
PO Box 890
Pacific Palisades CA 90272
(800) 459-3424   (310) 457-3811
Fax: (310) 457-0421   E-mail: simonton@lainet.com
Website: www.simontoncenter.com

Dr. Bernie Siegel
The Mind-Body Wellness Center
Meadville Medical Center
18201 Conneaut Lake Rd.
Meadville PA 16335
(814) 724-1765   Fax: (814) 333-8662
Website: www.mind-body.org

Deepak Chopra
The Chopra Center for Well Being
7630 Fay Ave.
La Jolla CA 92037
(888) 424-6772   (858) 551-7788
Fax: (858) 551-7811   E-mail: info@chopra.com
Website: www.chopra.com

Cancer Care

Commonweal
PO Box 316
Bolinas CA 94924   (415) 868-0970
Website: www.commonweal.org

Bristol Cancer Help Centre
Grove House
Cornwallis Grove, Clifton
Bristol BS8 4PG, UK
Centre information: +44-11-7980-9500
Helpline: +44-11-7980-9505
Website: www.bristolcancerhelp.org

Cancer and Cancer-Research Information

National Cancer Institute   (800) 4-CANCER (422-6237)
Website: www.cancer.gov

American Cancer Society   (800) ACS-2345
Website: www.cancer.org

American Institute for Cancer Research
(Focuses exclusively on the link between diet and cancer)
(800) 843-8114   E-mail: aicrweb@aicr.org
Website: www.aicr.org

Genetic Cancer Screening and Counseling

CancerNet (a service of the National Cancer Institute)

Cancer Genetics Services Directory
(an online list of professionals providing cancer genetics services)
Website: cancernet.nci.nih.gov/genesrch.shtml

Useful Organizations, Products, and Practitioners

Acupuncture

**National Certification Commission for Acupuncture
and Oriental Medicine**
(703) 548-9004
Website: www.nccaom.org

American Academy of Medical Acupuncture
(323) 937-5514
Website: www.medicalacupuncture.org
www.acupuncture.com

Alcoholism

Alcoholics Anonymous   (212) 870-3400
Website: www.aa.org

Bio-Energy Measuring

Scenar device (available from Life Energies, UK)
+44-17-2551-3129

Chi Gong (Qigong)

National Qigong Association   (218) 365-6330
E-mail: info@nqa.org
Website: www.nqa.org

Counseling

Association for Transpersonal Psychology
(415) 561-3382   E-mail: atpweb@mindspring.com
Website: www.atpweb.org

American Counseling Association
(703) 823-9800
Website: www.counseling.org/consumers_media

United Way Agencies
Check your local telephone directory.

Dowsing

The GEO Group
Website: www.geo.org/dowse1.htm

Electromagnetic Radiation Protection
(Including Mobile Phones)

RADAR Electromagnetic Stabilizer
(858) 793-9230   E-mail: info@radar3.com
Website: www.radar3.com

Growth and Personal Development

Association for Transpersonal Psychology
(415) 561-3382   E-mail: atpweb@mindspring.com
Website: www.atpweb.org

The Findhorn Foundation (UK)
+44-13-0969-0311 or -0880   E-mail: reception@findhorn.org
Website: www.findhorn.org

Healing the Emotions of the Past

Hoffman Quadrinity Process
(800) 506-5253   E-mail: hq@hoffmaninstitute.org
Website: www.hoffmaninstitute.org

The Order of Love (UK)   +44-20-7359-3000

Homeopathy

National Center for Homeopathy
(877) 624-0613   E-mail: info@homeopathic.org
Website: www.homeopathic.org

Massage

American Massage Therapy Association
(847) 864-0123
Website: www.amtamassage.org

Meditation

The Transcendental Meditation Program
(888) LEARN TM (532-7686)   E-mail: info@tm.org
Website: www.tm.org

Friends of the Western Buddhist Order
New York: (212) 932-0301   San Francisco: (415) 282-2018
(Call or e-mail for other U.S. locations)
E-mail: communications@fwbo.org
Website: www.fwbo.org

Menopause

FemGest Progesterone Cream
(800) 243-1791   E-mail: info@4progesterone.com
Website: www.4progesterone.com

Argyll Herbs (UK)
(suppliers of Menopausal Herb Formula, agnus castus, and black cohosh)
+44-19-3486-3353
Website: www.argyll-herbs.com.uk

Nutrition

Society of Certified Nutritionists   (800) 342-8037
Website: www.certifiednutritionist.com

American Association of Nutritional Consultants
(888) 828-2262
Website: www.aanc.net

American Dietetic Association   (312) 899-0040
Website: www.eatright.org

Price-Pottenger Nutrition Foundation
(800) FOODS-4-U (366-3748)   E-mail: info@price-pottenger.org
Website: www.price-pottenger.org

Overweight and Obesity

American Obesity Association   (800) 98-OBESE (986-2373)
Website: www.obesity.org

International Obesity Task Force
Website: www.iotf.org

Weight Watchers   (800) 651-6000
Website: www.weightwatchers.com

Overeaters Anonymous   (505) 891-2664
E-mail: info@overeatersanonymous.org
Website: www.overeatersanonymous.org

Radon

U.S. Environmental Protection Agency
National Radon Information Line: (800) SOS-RADON (767-7236)
Or, if you've already tested your home, the Radon FIX-IT Program:
(800) 644-6999
Website: www.epa.gov/iaq/radon
(provides radon contacts for each state as well as other extensive
information)

Relationship Problems

Human Awareness Institute   (800) 800-4117
E-mail: office@hai.org
Website: www.hai.org

Relaxation Tapes

Suki Productions   (877) 440-SUKI (440-7854)
E-mail: info@sukiproductions.com
Website: www.sukiproductions.com

Guided Imagery, Inc.   (440) 944-9292
Website: www.guidedimageryinc.com

Retreat Center

Vision Farms
PO Box 154
McIntosh FL 32664   (352) 591-4791
Fax: (352) 591-4898
Website: www.visionfarms.com

Namasté Retreat and Conference Center
29500 SW Grahams Ferry Rd.
Wilsonville OR 97070-9516   (800) 893-1000
Website: www.lecworld.org/Retreats.htm

Sacred Space Foundation (UK)   +44-17-8689-8375
E-mail: Jeannie@sacredspace.org.uk or Steve@sacredspace.org.uk
Website: www.sacredspace.org.uk

Shiatsu

American Oriental Body Therapy Association
(856) 782-1616   E-mail: aobta@prodigy.net
Website: www.aobta.org

Smoking

American Lung Association Freedom from Smoking Program
(Support groups are available in some states; the online program is open
to everyone.)
(800) LUNG USA (586-4872)   E-mail: info@lungusa.org
Website: www.lungusa.org/ffs/index.html

Spiritual Healing

World Light Center   (914) 297-2867
E-mail: healers@worldlightcenter.com
Website: www.worldlightcenter.com (offers an extensive online directory
of healers worldwide; inclusion in the directory requires no approval or
certification by World Light Center)

National Federation of Spiritual Healers (UK)
+44-19-3278-3164
E-mail: office@nfsh.org.uk
Website: www.nfsh.org.uk
www.silentunity.com

Tai Chi

International Taoist Tai Chi Society
(850) 224-5438 (U.S.)
(416) 656-2110 (Canada)
E-mail: (U.S.) usa@ttcs.org; (Canada) canada@ttcs.org
Website: www.taoist.org

Tantra

Tantra.com   (707) 823-3063
E-mail: questions@tantra.com
Website: www.tantra.com

Vitamin- and Mineral-Level Testing

Biolab Medical Unit (UK)
(offers a wide range of tests specifically looking at the effects of nutrition
and the environment on one's health; up to two-thirds of Biolab's tests
are available for U.S. customers)
+44-20-7636-5959
E-mail: info@biolab.co.uk
Website: www.biolab.co.uk

Tahoma Clinic   (253) 854-4900
E-mail: tahomac@tahoma-clinic.com
Website: www.tahomaclinic.com

Great Smokies Diagnostic Laboratories
(800) 522-4762   E-mail: cs@gsdl.com
Website: www.gsdl.com

Vitamins, Minerals, Herbs, and Plant Food Extracts

Bristol Cancer Help Centre Shop (UK)
+44-11-7980-9504

General Nutrition Centers (GNC)
For store locations or to order over the Internet, contact www.gnc.com

Specialty Products

Carctol
(available from Mrs. Yashu Amlani (UK), tel.: +44-11-7973-6052 or
from www.anticancerherb.com)

IP6 and MGN3 food concentrates
(available from the NutriCenter (UK), tel.: +44-20-7436-5122)

Yoga

Yoga Alliance
(877) YOGAALL (964-2255)   E-mail: info@yogaalliance.org
Website: www.yogaalliance.org

Tessa Morgan yoga tape
(audiotape for those limited physically; available from Bristol Cancer
Help Centre (UK))
+44-11-7980-9504)

Books

Cancer Prevention

Kune, Gabriel, M.D. *Reducing the Odds: A Manual for the Prevention of
Cancer.* St. Leonards, Australia: Allen and Unwin, 1999.

Anticancer Nutrition

Daniel, Rosy. *Healing Foods.* London: Thorsons Publishers, 1997.

Holford, Patrick. *Say No to Cancer.* London: Piatkus, 1999.

Holford, Patrick. *The Optimum Nutrition Bible.* Santa Cruz, CA: Crossing
Press, 1999.

Kenton, Leslie. *Raw Foods.* London: Vermillion, UK, 1998.

Olivier, Suzannah. *The Breast Cancer Prevention and Recovery Diet.* Wood-
land Publishing, 2001 [London: Penguin UK, 2000].

Olivier, Suzannah. *The Detox Manual.* New York: Simon and Schuster,
2001.

Plant, Jane A., Ph.D. *Your Life in Your Hands: Understanding, Preventing
and Overcoming Breast Cancer.* New York: St. Martins Press, 2000.

Healthy Cookbooks

Gavin, Paola. *Italian Vegetarian Cooking.* New York: M Evans & Co., 1994.

Jaffrey, Madhur. *Madhur Jaffrey's World Vegetarian.* New York: Clarkson
Potter, 2002.

Sen, Jane. *The Healing Foods Cookbook: The Vegan Way to Wellness.* London: Thorsons Publishers, 2001.

Sen, Jane. *More Healing Foods: Over 100 Delicious Recipes to Inspire Health and Wellbeing.* London: Thorsons Publishers, 2001.

Emotional and Spiritual Health

Bays, Brandon. *The Journey: A Road Map to the Soul.* New York: Pocket Books, 2001.

Breathnach, Sarah Ban. *Something More: Excavating Your Authentic Self.* New York: Warner Books, 2000.

Kübler-Ross, Elizabeth and David Kessler. *Life Lessons: Two Experts on Death and Dying Teach Us About the Mysteries of Life and Living.* New York: Scribner, 2000.

Pert, Candace B., Ph.D. *Molecules of Emotion: Why You Feel the Way You Feel.* New York: Simon & Schuster, 1999.

Household Carcinogens

Steinman, David, and Samuel S. Epstein, M.D. *The Safe Shopper's Bible.* New York: Hungry Minds, Inc., 1995.

The Holistic Approach to Cancer

Daniel, Dr. Rosy. *Living with Cancer.* London: Robinsons, UK, 2000.

Index

THE ART OF GETTING WELL: A Five-Step Plan for Maximizing Health When You Have a Chronic Illness

by David Spero, R.N., Foreword by Martin L. Rossman, M.D.

Self-management programs have become a key way for people to deal with chronic illness. In this book, David Spero brings together the medical, psychological and spiritual aspects of getting well in a five-step approach that asks you to slow down and use your energy for the things and people that matter; make small, progressive changes that build self-confidence; get help and nourish the social ties that are crucial for well-being; value your body and treat it with affection and respect; and take responsibility for getting the best care and health you can

224 pages ... Paperback $15.95 ... Hardcover $25.95

CHINESE HERBAL MEDICINE MADE EASY: Natural and Effective Remedies for Common Illnesses

by Thomas Richard Joiner

Chinese herbal medicine is an ancient system for maintaining health and prolonging life. This book demystifies the subject, with clear explanations and easy-to-read alphabetical listings of more than 750 herbal remedies for over 250 common illnesses ranging from acid reflux and AIDS to breast cancer, pain management, sexual dysfunction, and weight loss. Whether you are a newcomer to herbology or a seasoned practitioner, you will find this book a valuable addition to your health library.

432 pages ... Paperback $24.95 ... Hardcover $34.95

CANCER—INCREASING YOUR ODDS FOR SURVIVAL: A Resource Guide for Integrating Mainstream, Alternative and Complementary Therapies *by* David Bognar

This book provides a comprehensive look at traditional medical treatments for cancer and how these can be supplemented. It explains the basics of cancer and the best actions to take immediately after a diagnosis of cancer. It outlines the various conventional, alternative, and complementary treatments; describes the powerful effect the mind can have on the body and the therapies that strengthen this connection; and explores spiritual healing and issues surrounding death and dying. Includes full-length interviews with leaders in the field of healing, including Joan Borysenko, Stephen Levine, and Bernie Siegel.

352 pages ... Paperback $15.95 ... Hardcover $25.95

All prices subject to change

CANCER DOESN'T HAVE TO HURT: How to Conquer the Pain Caused by Cancer and Cancer Treatment

by Pamela J. Haylock, R.N., and Carol P. Curtiss, R.N.

People with cancer often suffer pain needlessly. Haylock and Curtiss show that not only can cancer pain be relieved, but patients who have less pain do better.

Readers learn how to describe their pain in specific terms that doctors understand, and ask for the pain relief they need. The authors also explain how to read prescriptions, administer medications, and adjust dosages if necessary. Also included are non-drug methods of pain relief that patients and caregivers can implement on their own, including massage, exercise, visual imagery, and music therapy.

192 pages ... 10 illus. ... Paperback $14.95 ... Hardcover $24.95

WOMEN'S CANCERS: How to Prevent Them, How to Treat Them, How to Beat Them — *Third edition in October 2002*

by Kerry A. McGinn, R.N. and Pamela J. Haylock, R.N.

This guide gives women detailed information on treating and surviving the cancers that exclusively affect them: breast, cervical, ovarian, uterine, and vaginal cancer, as well as lung and colon cancer. The second edition covers the latest screening guidelines and diagnostic tests, and the discovery of the breast cancer gene. The third edition will address late and long-term effects of cancer, the new FDA approved and "smart" drugs; and possible environmental factors in cancer development. The second edition will remain available till the new edition is released.

2nd edition: 512 pages ... 68 illus. ... Paperback $19.95 ... Hardcover $29.95
3rd edition: 560 pages ... 72 illus. ... Paperback $24.95 ... Hardcover $34.95

MEN'S CANCERS: How To Prevent Them, How To Treat Them, How To Beat Them

by Pamela J. Haylock R.N., M.A., E.T., Editor

This is a resource for men diagnosed with or concerned about cancer, their family members, and caregivers. Each chapter, written by a specialized nurse or nurse practitioner, covers prevention, early detection, diagnosis, treatments, follow-up, and recurrence. Special chapters address sex changes related to cancer and future directions in scientific research and study. An extensive resource section provides links to treatment centers, clinics, and helping organizations.

368 pp. ... 16 illus.... Paperback $19.95 ... Hardcover $29.95

To order see last page or call (800) 266-5592

THE PROSTATE HEALTH WORKBOOK: A Practical Guide for the Prostate Cancer Patient

by Newton Malerman, Foreword by Rachmel Cherner, M.D.

Each year over 180,000 men in the U.S. are diagnosed with prostate cancer. For those who survive, the journey toward recovery is often filled with worry, fear, and uncertainty.

Newton Malerman, a prostate cancer survivor, attributes his recovery to a proactive approach, and encourages readers to understand and fight the disease and get the best medical care possible.

Based on direct experience, extensive research and discussions with doctors, nurses, and other patients, he has written a hands-on book that includes 25 worksheets, from medical history checklists and treatment option evaluation charts to test result records.

160 pages ... 8 illus. 25 worksheets ... Paperback $14.95 ... Hardcover $24.95

THE FEISTY WOMAN'S BREAST CANCER BOOK

by Elaine Ratner.   ***Featured in The New York Times***

This personal, advice-packed guide helps women navigate the emotional and psychological landscape surrounding breast cancer, and make their own decisions with confidence. Its insight and positive message make this a perfect companion for every feisty woman who wants not only to survive but thrive after breast cancer.

"There are times when a woman needs a wise and level-headed friend, someone kind, savvy and caring... [This] book is just such a friend..." — Rachel Naomi Remen, M.D., author of *Kitchen Table Wisdom*

288 pages ... Paperback $14.95 ... Hardcover $24.95

LYMPHEDEMA: A Breast Cancer Patient's Guide to Prevention and Healing *by* Jeannie Burt and Gwen White, P.T.

This book emphasizes active self-help for lymphedema, the disfiguring and often painful swelling, particularly of the arm, that affects as many as 30 percent of breast cancer patients. It describes the many options women have for preventing and treating the condition, ranging from exercise to compression to massage.

"A very useful book for patients...a good practical resource for professionals."—Saskia J. Thiadens, R.N., Ex. Dir., National Lymphedema Network

224 pages ... 50 illus. ... Paperback $12.95 ... Hardcover $22.95

ORDER FORM

10% DISCOUNT on orders of $50 or more —
20% DISCOUNT on orders of $150 or more —
30% DISCOUNT on orders of $500 or more —
On cost of books for fully prepaid orders

NAME

ADDRESS

CITY/STATE   ZIP/POSTCODE

PHONE   COUNTRY (outside of U.S.)

TITLE	QTY	PRICE	TOTAL
The Cancer Prevention Book... (paperback)		@ $14.95	

Prices subject to change without notice

Please list other titles below:

		@ $	
		@ $	
		@ $	
		@ $	
		@ $	
		@ $	
		@ $	
		@ $	

Check here to receive our book catalog   ❏   free

Shipping Costs

First book: $3.00 by bookpost, $4.50 by UPS, Priority Mail, or to ship outside the U.S.
Each additional book: $1.00
For rush orders and bulk shipments call us at (800) 266-5592

TOTAL   _____
Less discount @____%   (_____)
TOTAL COST OF BOOKS   _____
Calif. residents add sales tax   _____
Shipping & handling   _____
TOTAL ENCLOSED   _____
Please pay in U.S. funds only

❏ Check ❏ Money Order ❏ Visa ❏ Mastercard ❏ Discover

Card # _____ Exp. date _____

Signature _____

Complete and mail to:
Hunter House Inc., Publishers
PO Box 2914, Alameda CA 94501-0914
Website: www.hunterhouse.com
Orders: (800) 266-5592 or email: **ordering@hunterhouse.com**
Phone (510) 865-5282 Fax (510) 865-4295

CPB — 3/2002